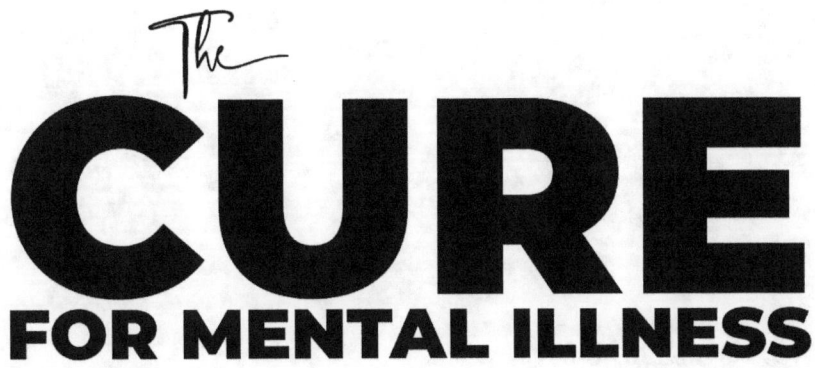

The CURE
FOR MENTAL ILLNESS

STAFF SERGEANT
PATRICK SIMS, RETIRED

ISBN 979-8-9891309-0-0

Copyright © 2023 by Aleah Jean Publishing

Printed in the United States of America

First Printing, 2023

Contents

Introduction 1

Section One: Awareness 7

    Anxiety Disorders 12

    Behavioral Disorders 19

    Eating Disorders 21

    Mood Disorders 23

    Suicidal Behavior 26

    Psychotic Disorders 28

Section Two: Understanding 33

Section Three: Perception 41

    Stigma and Discrimination:

        The Bane of Untreated Mental Illnesses 42

    Effects of Stigmatization 43

    How to Fight Stigmatization and

        Adopt a Positive Perception 44

Section Four: Support 47

    Psychotherapy 49

    Benefits of Psychotherapy 51

    Formats of Psychotherapy 53

    Types of Psychotherapy 54

Where Psychotherapy Can Help 59

How to Maximize Psychotherapy Sessions 60

Things to Consider Before Starting Therapy 61

How to Start Therapy 61

Alternative Treatments for Mental Health Illnesses 65

Models of Case Management 66

Natural Remedies 67

Support Groups 72

Complementary and Alternative Medicine 75

Things You Can Do to Improve Your Mental Health 83

How Does Self-help Affect Mental Health? 88

Why is Self-care Important? 92

Benefits of Self-Care 93

Section Five: Leap of Faith 95

Conclusion 99

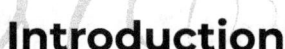

Introduction

What is mental health? There are plenty of complicated answers to that question. However, simply put, it is our emotional, psychological, and social well-being. How we think, handle stress, feel, act, make choices, and even relate to others are all products of our mental health. Your emotions, self-esteem, learning, communication, and relationships with people are all, therefore, influenced by it.

However, the brain is a part of the body, so biological changes and life experiences can affect your mental health. You may have developed mental health issues because of all kinds of things. Let's consider an example that involves post-traumatic stress disorder (PTSD). PTSD can be related to traumas, life experiences, and chemical factors.

Sarah, a military veteran, starts experiencing distressing nightmares, flashbacks, and intense anxiety after returning from active duty. She finds herself constantly on edge, avoiding places or situations that remind her of her traumatic experiences. She also notices a persistent negative shift in her mood and a loss of interest in activities she once enjoyed.

In this example, the development of PTSD is related to a traumatic event or events experienced during military service. Traumatic events can trigger changes in the brain and the body's stress response system, leading to the development of PTSD. The traumatic experience acts as the primary trigger for Sarah's mental health condition.

While the initial trauma is a significant factor, it's also essential to consider the interplay of other factors. Traumas alone may not explain why some individuals develop PTSD while others do not. Additional factors, therapy (or lack thereof) post-event is a factor, pre-existing vulnerabilities, social support, and coping skills, can influence the likelihood of developing PTSD.

Chemical factors also play a role. PTSD involves alterations to the brain's chemistry and neurobiology. Specifically, there may be imbalances in neurotransmitters (chemical messengers in the brain), such as serotonin and norepinephrine, which influence mood regulation and stress response. These chemical imbalances can contribute to the persistence and intensity of PTSD symptoms.

To sum it up, this example highlights how PTSD can be related to traumas (such as military experiences, childhood events, accidents), life circumstances (childhood abuse, job loss, death, divorce), and chemical factors. It underscores the complex interplay between environmental, psychological, and biological factors in the development of mental health conditions. It's important to approach mental health holistically, considering multiple factors when understanding and addressing mental illnesses.

Good mental health implies a state of balance where a person can effectively manage their emotions, handle stress, maintain positive relationships, and make rational choices. It involves having a sense of purpose, self-esteem, resilience, and the ability to adapt to change and cope with adversity.

The mind is a powerful thing. It can make or break you. So, why not protect it? If your memory has degraded, you have difficulty concentrating or have a feeling of uneasiness, please know that there are things you can do to help yourself get back on track.

The first step in addressing your mental illness is understanding what you need to do to reach an optimal level of awareness. **Awareness** is fundamental to any issue. Without it, we can't frame the issue and approach it from a healthy perspective. Gaining an understanding of what makes you tick from the right perspective will help you make sense of things. One way to gain awareness of factors that may be affecting your mental health is to take time to reflect on your thoughts, feelings, and behaviors. Consider any patterns or changes you have noticed in your mood, emotions, sleeping patterns, appetite, energy levels, or overall functioning. Pay attention to any persistent or significant difficulties or distress you may be experiencing.

Everyone has their own thought processes, and there are also subconscious aspects of the self that drive our thoughts and feelings. **Understanding** those helps one prioritize their time and resources based on their needs rather than those imposed by others. Don't forget that this is your illness and no one else's. For someone to even come close to fully understanding you, they would have to experience life and the pain that you have for themselves. Remember that understanding and treating your mental illness is a journey, and it may take time to gain clarity and develop a comprehensive plan. Be patient with yourself, practice self-compassion, and seek professional help where possible. Mental health professionals are trained to guide you through this process and provide you with the support you need.

Perception is vital. It is the filter through which we see the world, notice events, and interact with people. Perception drives our responses, which can be positive or negative and can determine if an event is merely a minor bump in the road or a major detour. Accurate perception of your mental illness increases the likelihood of seeking appropriate treatment. When you recognize that your symptoms align with a specific mental health condition, you are more likely to seek help.

In this context, **support** means having a support system of people in place so that while you're working on your internal struggles, they will believe in you, encourage you, and be on your side. Not being afraid to get help when necessary is essential for your recovery and growth. It shows that you're not afraid of taking care of yourself.

Lastly, a **leap of faith** involves putting trust in yourself and in your support system. It's about trusting that what we're doing is for the best, even though it might not always feel like it. Well, this is exactly what I'm talking about when it comes to getting help for your mental health. You need to trust that you are doing the right thing. Trust that people really want to help, and trust yourself and the decisions you make now that you are aware you need help.

There's no shame in admitting you need help—even if you're not sure what exactly it is you need help with—and there's no shame in seeking out a mental health professional. But I get it. It's hard to know where to start. Don't settle for someone who isn't right for you! Consider it a little like dating—keep looking until you find someone who makes you feel understood and cared for and can help guide you through this difficult time.

Mental health is one of the most important aspects of life. Without it, you'd just be a puddle of goo on the floor. And struggling with it is common. According to the National Alliance on Mental Illness, one in five adults has gone through or is currently going through some form of mental illness. Mood disorders affect almost 10% of adults each year, while PTSD affects over 18%.

Without identifying and understanding these issues, you won't be able to address them, and this will only result in more complications. Unprocessed pain produces self-sabotaging behavior.

Imagine you're walking down the street, minding your own business, and then, bam! You get hit by a car. It's not like you could have seen it coming; it just happened out of nowhere. Few people ever see the trauma they've experienced coming. Traumatic events generally occur out of nowhere and are often the result of some sort of crisis—ranging from the sinister to the mundane. The symptoms can range from mild to severe, and everyone deals with them in different ways and to varying degrees. Most people don't even realize how affected they are by trauma until much later in life (if at all). Because a person will know they have undergone a traumatic event, but may not know that it affected them.

Ever since I was a little kid, I've been fascinated by the idea of mental health. I would read any book that spoke about the human mind. Back then, growing up in poverty, I quickly learned that if your mind is right, you can survive anything. I mean, we all have moments when we feel like we're on top of the world… but what about when you don't feel like that? When you start to lose touch with reality and your own sense of self, that's when things get really scary.

But what if there were a way to make sure that never happened to you? I'm here to tell you there is.

"You cannot be great if you cannot operate in chaos [....] because if you can operate in chaos, the world becomes Disneyland, problems become scratches."
~ William Hollis

In this book, I'll share an overview my experience as an airman in Afghanistan, where I was deployed with SEAL Team IV, along with the lessons I learned there about mental health and the practice I received in helping people when I was a wounded warrior ambassador. You, too, can become whole again and live the life you truly deserve! You weren't created to live in penury or become a slave to your problems. You. Can. Overcome. Them.

This isn't a dry book of psychological theories, but one that contains solutions and methods through which you can attain optimal mental health, overcome mental challenges, and live soundly until your last day here on Earth.

Mental health issues are common, but solutions are available. You can get better many mental illnesses are incurable. They can be effectively managed with medication, therapy, and lifelong treatment First, you must comprehend the five elements to your path of recovery—awareness, understanding your problem, perception, support, and taking a leap of faith. These concepts, and many more, are explained in detail in the pages that follow.

Section One:

AWARENESS

Sure, you can try to make everyone happy. It's not going to work. You're human. They're human. You have different opinions, backgrounds, and values. And we all have problems. It's just part of being alive.

So, how do we deal with them? Well, there are two things you can do:

1. Be aware of your problems.
2. Take the initiative to solve them.

If you want to be successful in life—and who doesn't?—then facing your problems is a must. The only way out is through. Getting started solving your problems means being aware of them. And that means admitting you have them.

Mental health refers to someone's overall stability of mind and emotions. It is a combination of factors, such as a sense of purpose, self-esteem, personality, and thoughts. All these factors add up to our—hopefully positive—overall mental attitude towards life. Mental health challenges disrupt this stability and negatively affect daily functioning. Consequently, you not only become unable to work and function effectively, but also have trouble maintaining relationships with family and friends. There are also factors that can increase the risk of developing a mental disorder.

The cure to mental illness starts with being aware of your mental health. Awareness is vital to treatment because if you don't find out what's wrong with your health, you won't be able to find solutions. Awareness can help you understand the signs, and that's why it's the first step to curing mental illness in this book.

Awareness is all about knowing what is going on with you and what is going on around you. If you are aware of what your triggers or problems are, you are one step closer to finding the cure to your mental health. You will then be able to attack the problem from a better angle, and your situation will be less stressful. You should be able to know where that anxiety or depression is coming from. Is it connected to the past and perhaps related to where you grew up? If you are aware of your anxiety triggers, you won't turn around and falsely accuse other people of making you anxious. For instance, let's say you identify your anxiety trigger is junk food, you would feel guilty, and worried you'll gain weight, or contribute to an unhealthier body if they eat unhealthily? You then won't put the blame on others for triggering anxiety. This is why awareness is so important to solving mental health issues.

When I was 13 when I watched on national TV, Latasha Harlins get killed in a Korean store by Soon Ja Du, a 51-year-old Korean woman. Harlins was an African American, 15-year-old girl who just wanted to buy some orange juice. Soon Ja Du, one of the convenience store owners, thought she was trying to steal it and shot her in the back of the head.

This is one of the many examples of how I realized that people of color are treated differently than other people in our society. Can you imagine how a person's mental health is affected by racism? When Du was tried and convicted of voluntary manslaughter because of Harlin's death, her sentence was suspended. Instead, she was placed on five years probation with 400 hours of community service and made to pay $500 restitution and for Harlins' funeral expenses. If you're a Black man getting beat up by a group of racist cops… or a 15-year-old Black girl who just wants to buy some orange juice, you mean nothing.

The awareness of this injustice sparked riots throughout Los Angeles in 1992 after Martin Luther King Jr.'s "I Have a Dream" speech, as well as during desegregation efforts. Unfortunately, this is still happening today. There is an undertone and overtone of disdain and hatred toward the African American community because of racism, which has existed since slavery times but still endures to this day because we refuse to acknowledge it. Can you imagine being 13 years old and watching on TV that a 15-year-old girl got murdered while trying to buy some orange juice?

I learned about the plight of African Americans when I was 13 years old. I was just a kid, and I didn't really understand what was going on at the time.

But it was clear that something was wrong. I wasn't liked because I was Black, and that made me feel like something was wrong, too. But, as I look back and think about the incident now that I'm an adult, I am astonished. That was history being made and a life-changing moment, and I could relate to that. It helped negatively shape my behavior and mental health. It made me feel like my life as an African American did not matter. In the land of the "free", my people will not receive justice. Now, let's think about Natasha's family members and friends… what happened to them after the incident? How did it affect their mental health? Undoubtedly, they will live with that scar forever, as well as the stigma associated with the incident. This will have affected their mental health negatively. If they didn't seek therapy after her death, they may never have recovered from this heinous act committed against their daughter/sister/mother/friend/etc.

When the store owner was not patient enough to understand what Natasha was doing, she ended up swimming in her own blood and being buried six feet under. This story really cements the importance of being aware of the things happening in your environment, as you will then have a better chance of addressing the problem without complicating it. If the Soon Ja Du, the wife of the convenience store owner had been patient enough to find out what the Black girl was doing in her store, Natasha would still be with us.

This also applies to mental health. If you have issues with your mental health, you need to first identify what's happening to you before addressing it. Be patient with yourself and with others.

Mental illnesses are more common than you think. In fact, close to 19% of adults, 46% of teenagers, and 13% of children are affected by mental health issues every year. It's no surprise that teenagers are most affected since most life-changing experiences occur at this stage of life.

People suffering from mental illness may be your neighbors, may attend the same church as you, or may be your colleague at work. If you are not aware of the problems you have, you will have a difficult time addressing them and understanding those of others. How can you become aware of your problems? How can you identify the factors responsible for your sudden mood changes, vindictiveness, or spontaneous irrational behaviors? First, let's look at the types of mental illnesses:

Types of Mental Illness

People can experience different mental illnesses that may affect their thinking, how they relate to other people, and their moods and behaviors. You need to become aware of the various forms of these mental health problems so that you can fight them using the right channels. Let's look at the different types.

Anxiety Disorders

Anxiety can be defined as a feeling of worry, nervousness, or uneasiness. It's a normal human emotion that everyone experiences from time to time. Anxiety disorders, on the other hand, are characterized by persistent and irrational fear in situations where there is no danger or threat present. An anxiety disorder can lead to severe problems in daily life, such as loss of sleep, reduced performance at work or school, and an overall feeling of helplessness.

Anxiety disorders are further categorized into post-traumatic stress disorder (PTSD), obsessive-compulsive Disorder (OCD), panic disorders, and phobias. I will briefly discuss anxiety and anxiety disorders, as well as their subtypes, symptoms, and causes.

Anxiety disorders are prevalent, so much so that they are the most common type of mental disorder and affect about 18% of the US population. A research study conducted by Cambridge University concluded that anxiety disorders are more common in women than men, with women being twice as likely to be affected by one. People under 35 years of age are more likely to experience an anxiety disorder than any other group. People diagnosed with terminal illnesses such as cancer or chronic diseases and diabetes are also at an elevated risk of having an anxiety disorder. In terms of worldwide statistics, 4 out of every 100 people suffer from an anxiety disorder, with Asia having the lowest average rate of 3 in 100 and North America having the highest average rate of 8 in 100. People diagnosed with anxiety disorders are three to five times more likely to seek help from a therapist, and six times more likely to be hospitalized in a psychiatric facility.

Anxiety disorders also affect a person's mental health more broadly, as they are often associated with depression. There is a considerable overlap in the number of people with anxiety disorders also being diagnosed with depression. When two or more mental illnesses are present, these are called co-occurring disorders.

Anxiety Disorders

Anxiety disorders prevent people from doing many things, including concentrating and just going about their day normally. There are six types of anxiety disorders:

Generalized Anxiety Disorder (GAD)

GAD affects 3.1% of the US population and is often associated with major depression. GAD is characterized by uncontrollable worrying about events and activities that may result in a negative outcome. A person diagnosed with GAD is often disturbed by that worry and anxiety. His/her daily life, social life, academic life, and ability to function are all affected.

Symptoms of GAD include excessive worry, difficulty concentrating and studying, and an inability to socialize. Other symptoms, like depression and headaches because of drug and alcohol abuse, can also be present. Symptoms must persist for six months or longer before a person can be diagnosed with GAD.

GAD is often caused by a combination of factors, which may include:

- Biological - includes some changes in the functioning of the amygdala in the brain.
- Psychological - being overly sensitive, over-analyzing situations, and being extremely nervous.
- An Event or Incident - particularly stressful events, such as a

trauma, can change a person's way of life and can trigger GAD. Examples of these events include sexual abuse, a break-up, losing a job, the death of a child, etc.

- Genetics - a close relative with a history of mental health problems can pass GAD onto a close blood relative.

Obsessive-Compulsive Disorder (OCD)

OCD is a common anxiety disorder among both men and women that affects about 2.2 million adults in the U.S. OCD symptoms will present at an early age and continue to affect children into their adulthood. A person with OCD has persistent thoughts and will often obsess over thoughts and/or events, which causes them immense distress. Someone with OCD will attempt to solve these problems by performing sets of repetitive, specific actions. A person with OCD feels that any change in this ritualistic way of performing certain tasks will inflict self-harm or affect others negatively. An example of this would be a person who forgets to do something important and may feel concerned that such forgetfulness will lead to a disproportionately bad outcome. A person who constantly checks if their money is missing from their pockets is a common example of compulsions. Compulsions like this don't necessarily mean these people have OCD, though. For OCD to be diagnosed, more than one symptom needs to be present.

Symptoms of OCD include:

- Intense, debilitating fear.
- Rapid breathing.
- Insomnia.
- Nervousness.

Post-Traumatic Stress Disorder (PTSD)

Globally, women are more likely to be affected by PTSD than men. Many things can trigger the development of PTSD. Rape, the unexpected death of a loved one, a violent incident, and accidents are all common triggers. Statistically, 65% of men and 46% of women who are raped will develop PTSD.

A person suffering from PTSD involuntarily recounts traumatic experiences (commonly called flashbacks), and this is accompanied by debilitating fear and a feeling of panic. These symptoms are especially severe if such situations present themselves again.

Symptoms of PTSD include:

- Deliberately avoiding people associated with events - the person avoids any kind of reminder of the event because it brings back excruciating memories.
- Insomnia - the person cannot sleep and may have recurring nightmares that disrupt their sleep.
- Mood changes – the person is irritated and is constantly on high alert for any sign of danger. This often occurs around the same time of day when the incident occurred.
- Inability to concentrate - whether at school, home or at work, the person is unable to concentrate on any activity. They are too absorbed in flashbacks.

Other symptoms include sweating, panic attacks, crippling fear, and stuttering.

Panic Disorder

Panic disorder does not require a specific trigger to develop in a person. It is an out-of-the-blue disorder and is associated with sudden panic attacks. Panic disorder seldom has a lasting effect on an individual, and most times, panic attacks last for a few minutes to an hour.

Symptoms of panic disorder include rapid breathing, profuse sweating, and trembling.

Social Disorder

A small percentage of the world's population suffer from disorders of this type. Social anxiety disorder varies in severity from person to person and is characterized by the fear of interacting or socializing with unfamiliar people. Such persons feel socially imprisoned and reserved to such an extent that they may avoid going to work, going to class, or any social gatherings entirely. A socially disordered individual experiences discomfort during social contact. Imposing certain restrictions to accommodate their disorder by minimizing social interaction is a common manifestation of this disorder.

A person suffering from this disorder ensures that similar encounters with unfamiliar people are not repeated because of fear. To an extent, they have difficulty interacting with people of different social stratifications. Examples of this include those of other races, genders, and classes. These feelings are common among young people and usually stay with them into adulthood. Social anxiety disorder can be associated with stranger anxiety disorder in the sense that unfamiliar people are involved.

Common symptoms of social anxiety disorder include stammering when on the verge of speaking, and perspiring profusely. The person is afraid that others will notice the symptoms mentioned above. Hence, they restrain from socializing. They worry they will be made fun of by people if they say or do something wrong, embarrassing, or humiliating. As you might guess, social anxiety disorder can affect both personal and professional relationships negatively. Other symptoms include trembling, nausea, and even diarrhea.

Typical symptoms must be present for at least six months for one to be diagnosed with this disorder. Effects of these symptoms include stress, social avoidance, and avoidance of routine activities.

There are several reasons why social anxiety disorder can manifest, including:

- Environment - this plays a huge part in the development of an anxiety disorder. If you are a victim of bullying in school, for example, then the chance of developing this disorder later in life is heightened.
- Genetics - it can run in a family, and there is a high possibility that it has developed phenotypically.
- Behavioral habits - a child or an adolescent who is shy, clingy, timid, or regularly crying is likely to develop this disorder in adulthood. Being overwhelmed by the person you are going to meet or an event you are going to attend for the first time can cause temporal social disorder. It is called temporal because it usually disappears after meeting such persons or attending that particular event.

Specific Phobias

A person with this anxiety disorder may have certain concerns or fears about a specific situation, activity, or animal. Such persons may feel anxious when they encounter a snake, or when traveling on a plane for the first time, or when climbing. The rational response to this is fear, because these situations or animals can pose a threat to his/her safety.

Some people, however, react by imagining danger that is blown out of proportion when exposed to certain situations or activities, even though that situation or activity is safe. Out of panic and fear, they are terrorized and feel disproportionately afraid. Sometimes, the mere thought or the sight of whatever they have a phobia of on the TV is enough to trigger a phobic reaction. These types of excessive reactions may be indicative of a specific phobia.

Specific phobias are often interrelated with panic attacks. Hence, they share the same symptoms—dizziness, chest pain, and other physical sensations.

The following factors are likely to increase the chance of developing a specific phobia:

- Genetics - specific phobias like a fear of spiders (arachnophobia) and fear of enclosed spaces (claustrophobia) may run in the family. If you have witnessed someone being bitten by an animal or have been bitten by one yourself, you may genuinely fear for your life if you subsequently see one of those animals.
- Environment - for example, if a person is used to living somewhere with many ground-level buildings, they may develop acrophobia, the fear of heights, when moving to a high-rise building. Sometimes, constant interaction and familiarity can reduce this disorder.

Separation Anxiety Disorder

This disorder manifests when an individual experiences anxiety due to separation from home, or from people with whom they have a strong emotional connection with. Children typically suffer from this anxiety disorder between the ages of six months and seven years old. It can also manifest in older children. This type of disorder is characterized by the separation of one person from another. Separation of a child from his mother, for example, can trigger this disorder. Depending on the type of person, this disorder may remain with the person for a lifetime. Separation anxiety disorder shows a certain form of cognitive maturity in children as they develop, so it shouldn't necessarily be interpreted as a behavioral problem.

Symptoms of separation anxiety disorder include:

- Clinginess - children with separation anxiety experience more disturbances and face greater obstacles in their academic development than those who do not have the disorder. They are disruptive in class and may refuse to attend school at first. Children protest on arrival and have a hard time saying good-bye to their parents. This attitude wears out as the child adjusts to the school setting.

- Fear of being alone - people—mostly children—who have this disorder have problems staying alone in a particular place. This is worsened if the environment is dark.

- Difficulty concentrating - this applies to both adults and children. Separation anxiety disorder makes it difficult for people to concentrate on their activities. They are consumed with their feelings and concerns about the environment and the people they left behind. Hence, productivity is reduced.

A combination of biological, environmental, and behavioral factors contributes to the development of separation anxiety disorder. Circumstances, such as losing a loved one, a change of school, or a change of residence, can trigger separation anxiety disorder.

Separation anxiety disorder may be heritable. It is estimated that separation anxiety disorder is more common in girls than in boys. In some instances, temperament also plays a role. A more timid child may be prone to developing this disorder.

Agoraphobia

Agoraphobia is a disorder characterized by fear of an environment which is perceived as unsafe and from which there is no easy means of escape. A person with this disorder experiences symptoms similar to panic attacks. This disorder may result in the sufferer staying at home all the time.

Open spaces and large locations, such as a bus or train station, are all situations that can trigger this disorder. Traumatic events such as the death of a loved one or a close relation may be a trigger. Agoraphobia is often associated with other anxiety disorders, such as specific phobias, separation disorder, and social anxiety disorder. The condition is less common in old age, and usually will first present itself in early adulthood. Women are twice as likely as men to experience it.

Symptoms of agoraphobia draw many parallels with panic disorder, social anxiety disorder, and separation anxiety disorder symptoms. Perceived fear is usually the most common symptom. The sufferer is constantly afraid of large, outdoor locations and has difficulty leaving their home and venturing outside of their comfort zone.

Agoraphobia is caused by a combination of genetic and environmental factors. Stressful events often contribute to the development of agoraphobia. Sufferers have an attachment issue because they can't tolerate a place outside their comfort base. Long-term use of alcohol and drugs like benzodiazepines can cause agoraphobia.

Behavioral Disorders

Behavioral disorders make up a pattern of "zigzag" behaviors. They are common in children and can last for up to six months. These behaviors involve a series of disruptive actions that can cause them problems in school, at home, and during social functions. Behavioral disorders include attention-deficit hyperactivity disorder (ADHD), oppositional defiant disorder (ODD), and conduct disorder. Behavioral disorders may include inattention, hyperactivity, impulsivity, drug use, defiant behavior, and criminal tendencies.

ADHD

Attention-deficit hyperactivity disorder (ADHD) is the most common behavioral disorder. It includes being unable to focus, being hyperactive when it comes to doing unimportant things, and being unable to control behaviors. ADHD usually starts in childhood, before progressing into adulthood. It's more common in boys than girls. A combination of genes and environmental factors play key roles in the development of ADHD. According to brain scans, the brains of people with ADHD work differently to those without the condition.

The signs of ADHD are pretty obvious and are divided into three categories: inattentive, hyperactivity, and impulsivity signs. One child with ADHD may show hyperactivity symptoms, while others may have only the other two. Inattentive symptoms include failure to pay close attention to detail, finding it hard to follow instructions and finish home tasks or school assignments in a timely manner, organizational problems, forgetfulness, and high levels of distractibility.

Hyperactivity symptoms include squirming while sitting, running about excessively, having issues playing normally, always being on the go with no clear destination in mind, talking excessively, and fidgeting.

Impulsivity signs include difficulty awaiting turns in queues, frequently interrupting conversations, and blurting out answers to questions before they are fully asked.

Eating Disorders

A person suffering from an eating disorder may have an uncontrollable appetite that results in them gaining considerable weight. On the other hand, a person with this disorder could have a negative attitude towards food, so that they feel eating will make them become fatter than they already are, even though they are thin. The most common eating disorders are anorexia nervosa, binge eating disorder, and bulimia.

Anorexia Nervosa

Anorexia nervosa makes people want to lose more weight than what is healthy for their age and height. In other words, people with this disorder are afraid of gaining weight, even when they are already underweight. They may diet excessively, engage in rigorous weight loss exercise, or use other unconventional methods to achieve their so-called "goal".

The cause of this type of eating disorder is unknown, but genes and social attitudes could play a role. If such a person regularly watches advertisements that promote slim body types, they may be determined to make theirs look the same. Risk factors for this disorder include paying unnecessary attention to body weight, having a negative self-image, having issues with food during childhood, trying to be overly perfect, and having certain kinds of social perspectives about health and beauty.

How do you know if you have anorexia nervosa? This mental health issue is more common in goal-oriented females than males. If you have an intense fear of gaining weight even when you are underweight, are focused on body weight so much that you think about other things less, exercise compulsively regardless of the circumstances you are in, or use pills to reduce your appetite, these are signs you may be suffering from anorexia nervosa.

Other signs include blotchy skin, confusion, depression, increased sensitivity to cold, and feelings of inferiority, especially when you see someone with what you deem to be a "perfect" body on the TV, social media, or in a magazine.

Binge Eating Disorder

Another type of eating disorder is binge eating. This is slightly different to anorexia nervosa because here, the person eats excessively during short intervals—much higher portions than a typical person of their size and weight does. When binge eating, the individual has the urge to continue eating, with no control over how much or how quickly they eat. This eating disorder usually leads to obesity. How do you know if you are suffering from binge eating?

While we can't really pinpoint the causes of this type of eating disorder, the warning signs are obvious. A binge eater consumes up to 15,000 calories in one meal, often eats snacks, and sweats profusely. Binge eating may co-occur with disorders like bulimia.

Bulimia

Bulimia is similar to binge eating disorder. The person has a loss of control over their eating and eats frequently, and will purge their meal by making themselves vomit or abusing laxatives to prevent weight gain. Like anorexia nervosa, it's more common in women than men, especially amongst adolescent girls and younger women. The exact cause of bulimia is unknown but may be genetic or psychological.

How do you realize that you have this disorder? Interestingly, most people suffering from this disorder are aware of their abnormal eating patterns and may even feel guilty about it, but they do nothing to resolve the issue, thus continuing with their unhealthy eating and purging habit. The key sign of this disorder is eating excessively at short intervals, followed by going to the bathroom to purge the food and prevent digestion.

Mood Disorders

Sometimes called affective disorders, mood disorders involve abnormal changes in mood. A person's mood may rapidly fluctuate between extreme joy and sadness. Most times, the individual feels down and sad, and feels the world is against them. As a result, the person loses interest in life. Mood disorders can be grouped into depression, bipolar disorder, seasonal affective disorder (SAD), and self-harm.

Depression

Depression is a state of unhappiness or low morale, which lasts for several days to weeks, months, or even years. The depressive individual visualizes an unhappy future and doesn't enjoy the moment. Over 20 million Americans suffer from depression, making it one of the most prevalent mental illnesses in the country. Depression doesn't go away easily, especially if the triggers are still present, and can substantially interfere with daily functioning.

A depressive person is sad, has a loss of interest in activities that they normally enjoy, develops insomnia, feels worthless, and may even have thoughts of committing suicide. Depression is a disorder of the brain that can be caused by a wide range of genetic, psychological, environmental, and biochemical factors.

Bipolar Disorder

Bipolar is a brain disorder that causes changes in a person's mood, energy levels, and ability to function at their optimal mental capacity. It involves having disoriented emotional states that occur at certain periods of the day or week, known as episodes. These episodes are categorized into manic, hypomanic, and major depressive episodes. A person with bipolar disorder has mood fluctuations that can last for hours, or days, or weeks. These swings can hugely disrupt a person's ability to form and maintain relationships, attend school or work, and stay safe.

The causes of bipolar disorder remain unclear, but it's believed that an imbalance of brain chemicals can lead to irregular brain functioning. Bipolar also disorder runs in families, and 80% to 90% of individuals with bipolar disorder may also experience depression, an anxiety disorder, ADHD, and develop suicidal thoughts. However, suicidal thoughts are more common with people with bipolar I than bipolar II. Mood swings can be triggered by stress, sleep disruption, and alcohol.

Let's talk about bipolar episodes. People with bipolar I disorder are often diagnosed when they experience manic, hypomanic, and major depressive episodes. Manic episodes last a period of around one week. When a person is irritable or seems to be overly energetic, it's a sign that they are having a manic episode. That person may experience insomnia, talk faster than usual, have uncontrollable racing thoughts, get distracted more easily, appear restless or highly spirited, and engage in risky behaviors, such as shopping sprees.

If these behaviors deviate from the person's usual behavior and are severe enough to disrupt the person's work and other regular activities, such a person will be diagnosed with bipolar. An individual experiencing manic episodes may also hallucinate and have disorganized thinking.

Hypomanic episodes are less severe manic symptoms. They typically last for four days, and the symptoms do not hinder one's daily activities, unlike manic episodes. Major depressive episodes typically last for two weeks or more. The person has the following symptoms: despair, loss of interests, guilt, tiredness, insomnia/increased sleep, lack of appetite, and suicidal thoughts.

Bipolar II disorders are diagnosed if the patient experiences some symptoms of major depressive and hypomanic episodes.

Seasonal Affective Disorder (SAD)

Some people have mood swings during winter, while others behave differently during fall. The series of abnormal changes due to weather can make a person feel sad, pessimistic, and restless. This condition is called seasonal affective disorder (SAD).

Seasonal affective disorder is a form of depression, known as major depressive disorder with seasonal pattern. Symptoms of SAD typically occur in the fall and winter period because of the lack of sunlight. While SAD is common in fall and winter, people can also experience it in summer, but that is rare. In the United States, about 5% of adults experience SAD, and it's more common in women than men.

SAD is proven to be a product of a biochemical imbalance in the brain, instigated by shorter hours of daylight and longer hours of darkness. As winter approaches, a shift in the circadian rhythm of the brain occurs, which makes people miscalculate their schedules. Although many people have adapted to these weather changes, some still find it hard to adjust. Symptoms of SAD can range from mild to severe.

How do you know if you have SAD? Symptoms include sadness, anxiety, feelings of being "empty," irritability, low energy, insomnia, weight changes, weight gain due to excessive carbohydrate consumption, engaging in purposeless activities such as pacing, difficulty making decisions, and feeling guilty. People with SAD often prefer to stay at home all day or all week, prompting them to eat excessively. Suicidal thoughts can also arise, especially if the sufferer is lonely.

Self-Harm

Self-harm is a severe form of mood disorder. It entails harming oneself intentionally by cutting, punching, pulling out hair, or burning oneself. It's more common in females than males and affects one in a hundred people. Most times, this individual has no intention of killing him or herself (in some cases, suicide may occur), instead, they do this to inflict injury upon themselves. Some people stop the act after a few occurrences, but others may have difficulty stopping themselves. Subsequent acts can result in higher risks of attempted suicide if the person doesn't get help.

Many people involved in these acts do it for the sense of relief. The pain derived from cutting their skin often gives them a sense of comfort. Some people also do this to cope with a difficult situation. Many teens have confessed to engaging in these self-harm acts to take their minds off a bad situation, such as to stop intrusive thoughts of guilty or feeling lonely and angry. This is why the condition is more common in teens and younger adults.

Suicidal Behavior

Suicidal behavior is a common mental health problem in the world today. Statistically, about 132 Americans die every day by suicide, making it the second leading cause of death among 15-24-year-olds. In addition, over 9.4 million adults in the United States have had thoughts about committing suicide in the past year.

Why do people resort to suicidal behavior? What are the signs that you have this mental illness so you can address it early? Obviously, it becomes apparent that someone is on the verge of committing suicide if they talk about killing themselves, but also if they talk about how hopeless they are, openly confess to feeling trapped or being a burden to others when they are clearly not, are unnecessarily agitated, and have increased their use of alcohol or drugs. Other signs include sleeping too much or too little, staying isolated, anger, mood swings, and talking about revenge.

It's crucial to note that suicidal thoughts can also arise as a result of an untreated mental illness. For instance, suicidal ideation, as it is sometimes called, can manifest if one has bipolar disorder, depression, schizophrenia, or substance use disorder. Those who have PTSD or who have experienced a traumatic event are also at a higher risk of committing suicide. The risk is elevated if their family has a history of suicide or suicidal ideation.

Suicide is scary, and the risk is dire for people who exhibit suicidal behavior. People with mental illnesses and who struggle with addiction have a higher chance of contemplating suicide. This is because drugs and alcohol affect thinking patterns, and when taken in large quantities can result in risky behaviors and reckless decision making.

Now, there's a difference between active suicidal ideation and passive suicidal ideation. The fundamental difference is intent. In passive ideation, the thoughts are there, but you have no intent to execute them. For example, you could say, "I wish I was dead." But when it comes to active ideation, the thoughts are there, and you have crafted a plan for how to kill yourself.

For instance, someone may say they are going to commit suicide, research methods, or write a suicide letter.

Psychotic Disorders

Psychotic disorders are mental disorders that cause abnormal thinking. They are serious illnesses that affect the mind and make it difficult for someone to think logically, communicate well, and behave appropriately. People with psychosis lose touch with reality and often hallucinate.

Delusions are another common symptom of this disorder and involve false perceptions, such as hearing and seeing things that are not really there. People with other types of mental illness, such as bipolar and anxiety disorder, may also experience psychotic symptoms.

The common types of psychotic disorders include schizophrenia, schizoaffective disorder, schizophreniform disorder, brief psychotic disorder, delusional disorder, and paraphrenia.

Schizophrenia

Schizophrenia is a type of psychotic disorder that manifests as delusions and hallucinations. It lasts for more than six months and can seriously affect relationships and concentration. This mental disorder starts in the teens to early 30s. Although this disorder affects both men and women, men tend to get it earlier. While men get diagnosed in their late teens, women are diagnosed in their late 20s to early 30s. Schizophrenia affects about 1% of the world's population. In the U.S., it affects about 3.5 million people.

Schizophrenia is difficult to diagnose, because people with this mental illness aren't usually aware that they are ill. In addition, the changes leading to schizophrenia can mirror those of normal life changes, so the patient and those around them assume nothing is wrong. For example, an affected teen might take up with some new friends or stop visiting their old pals. These are normal changes, but no one will question why that person is suddenly hanging out with new friends or has stopped visiting the ones they have known all their lives.

Schizophrenia can develop later in life, too. People over the age of 45 can be diagnosed as late-onset, with typical symptoms like delusions and hallucinations. These people are less likely to be diagnosed with other symptoms. Genetics are the major cause of this late-onset subtype. In younger children, this disorder may be diagnosed if their school performance drops drastically, or they avoid spending time with family and friends, are depressed, have no motivation, display odd behaviors, or walk unusually.

How do you know if someone has schizophrenia? Signs of schizophrenia are the general symptoms of psychotic disorders. Common signs include difficulty sleeping, hallucinations, delusions, paranoia, disordered thinking, and movement disorders or catatonia. Some of the major causes of psychosis include drug use, brain tumors, and stroke. Some of these things are self-inflicted, while others are medical conditions.

Schizoaffective Disorder

People who have the symptoms of mood disorders like depression and schizophrenia, are sometimes diagnosed with schizoaffective disorder. This disorder is a chronic mental health condition that is sometimes initially misdiagnosed as bipolar disorder. Doctors are uncertain if this condition is related to schizophrenia or mood disorder, but it is usually treated as a combination of both conditions.

Only a tiny percentage of the population is affected by this disorder (about 0.03%). It affects both men and women but is more common in women. It usually begins between the ages of 16 and 30 and is uncommon in children.

Schizoaffective disorder is either of the bipolar type or depressive type. Symptoms are nearly the same, and include delusions, sadness, worthlessness, hallucinations, lack of personal care, racing thoughts, sudden outbursts of unusual behavior, speech and communication problems, and difficulty concentrating. This disorder often runs in the family, or is caused by brain structure abnormalities, environmental factors, or drug use.

Schizophreniform Disorder

This disorder shares similar symptoms with schizophrenia, but they last for a shorter time—between one and six months. A person with schizophreniform disorder can't tell the difference between reality and imagination. The disorder affects how the person thinks, acts, expresses their emotions, and relates to others. About one in a thousand people develop this mental condition. It's more common in men than women, especially between the ages of 18 and 24. In women, it typically occurs between the ages of 24 and 35.

Brief Psychotic Disorder

People with this condition will experience a brief period of psychotic behavior, usually in response to a stressful event. Psychotic disorders come in three different forms. The first of which is brief psychotic disorder with an obvious stressor, which happens shortly after a trauma, such as losing someone close. The other two forms are brief psychotic disorder without a stressor and brief psychotic disorder with postpartum onset. The latter happens to a mother after four weeks of having a baby. People typically recover from this medical condition in less than a month.

Delusional Disorder

A person who holds false beliefs or the notion that he/she is in danger is known to be delusional. An affected individual will find it hard to believe that something isn't true. The person will have a false idea, experience, or memory, and then cling to it, to the extent that they say it all the time and firmly believe it actually happened or is the truth.

Delusional disorder is divided into mood, perception, memory, and ideas. In mood, the person has a strange feeling that the world they live in is odd and threatens their existence. In perception delusion, the individual feels that what they believe in is real, while most times, it isn't. With memory, the person has an inaccurate recollection of events, and in ideas, the affected individual forms thoughts out of nowhere.

Paraphrenia

A person suffering from this condition shares similar symptoms with schizophrenia. This condition is more commonly diagnosed in the elderly as opposed to other age groups.

General Signs of Mental Illness

If you experience the following behavioral changes, it's possible that you could be suffering from mental illness:

- Eating excessively or having no appetite.
- Sleeping too much or too little.
- Having low energy.
- Always feeling numb.
- Smoking and drinking excessively.

- Feeling confused, angry, worried, or scared of a perceived danger.
- Engaging in unnecessary fights and arguments.
- Hearing voices or seeing things that aren't there.
- Believing in things that aren't true.
- Thinking of harming others or yourself.
- Inability to concentrate at work or school, etc.

The first step in dealing with mental illness is being aware of the symptoms. These are not just "in your head", they're real, and they can have devastating effects on your life if left untreated.

The good news is that there are treatments out there for you! Keeping your symptoms to yourself will only make things worse for you and those close to you. This is why awareness is so vital. Apart from helping you understand the various mental illness symptoms, it can help you identify the resources available to treat them, and break the stigma associated with these issues.

Having a mental disorder doesn't mean you are inferior or crazy. Learn your weaknesses so you can turn them into strengths. To be effective in life, you must be willing to face difficult problems. Pretending that everything in your world is perfect is only going to lead to problems. It took me three years to be able to sit in the passenger seat of a car. I use that fear as a stepping stone to face my problems. I used to say that it was hard facing my PTSD, but now I say that it's easy, but just hard to put into practice. Admitting you have problems, then moving quickly to find solutions, is the key to success. Section four will discuss the treatment options available and how you can access them.

Section Two:

UNDERSTANDING

There's a method to everyone's madness, and there's a "why" for everything that happens. So, if you understand why you are experiencing triggers, a relapse, suicidal thoughts, or PTSD, it will help you overcome that mental illness and be less upset with people and your life. If those people understand what you are going through, they will understand how to relate to you better.

Let me share some of my story with you. I have been in the military for a while, but the thing that always blows my mind is how much you can learn from other people.

I was deployed as part of the SEAL IV team to Afghanistan in 2011. Then, the air force was helping the army in a joint operation. I was moved from one unit to the other, because each unit didn't need me. They said they didn't know who I was, and that they weren't expecting me. Finally, I was told to watch over the village cooks and take inventory somewhere in the Kandahar province, since I knew a few things about cooking. The intention was to prevent the villagers from poisoning the soldiers. I was responsible for monitoring supply shipments, gunships, supply drops, and was in charge of convoys. You know, that real high-octane and adrenaline pumping G.I. Joe stuff! Basically, I was in charge of transportation.

I was deployed to Afghanistan for seven months, but it felt like seven years. I came home and was supposed to go back to work after a month. However, I wasn't able to contact anyone in my unit. I tried to call them, but none of the numbers my command gave me worked.

I had to stay an extra month in Afghanistan and travel with the SEAL team. On my way out, I intended to drop off my armor, because it was mandated that it didn't leave the country. I met with a sergeant and told him my reason for coming—to leave my armor with him—and he told me to hold off for a second so he could check the system for identification. To my astonishment, he told me my name wasn't there… the military didn't know that I'd been deployed in the first place. I could have died out there and would have been forgotten because I wasn't being tracked. I had a death stare on my face when he told me this. To put it lightly, I was upset. His response was, "You'd be amazed at how many times this happens." As I was leaving his office, I remember seeing a sign on his door that said, "No airman left behind this is our job."

The war in Afghanistan was responsible for my PTSD, and I needed to understand that.

I couldn't sleep on the bed or sit down in the passenger seat of a vehicle for three years. While I was in Afghanistan, I injured my ankle and ripped the ligament out. No one truly understood what I was going through, and I didn't understand why I was finding it difficult to sleep. The noises from the gunshots that were playing in my head, and everything else, had left me traumatized and angry, and I began to develop PTSD.

Applying the "why" here, you will comprehend that my PTSD resulted from the conflict I experienced and witnessed, and the lack of support. The recollections of the conflict latched onto my subconscious mind and were left untreated. Understanding that the conflict was responsible for my PTSD helped me finally beat my psychological instability.

I'll explain the steps I took in Section Four.

Research has shown that mental health issues are caused by a variety of factors. The major ones are environment, genes, brain structure/chemistry, psychology/trauma, and occupation. Let's break down these factors and explain how each one of them can cause a mental health disorder.

1. The Environment

Environment plays a huge role in a person's behavior. If an individual spent most, or even part of their childhood in a violent neighborhood, their chances of becoming violent are high. Such a person could easily become an arms dealer, drug dealer, or may go on to orchestrate gang robberies. On the other hand, if they grew up in an area that was violence-free, the odds that they would become a menace are close to zero.

A pregnant mother exposed to certain stressors—inflammatory conditions, alcohol, poor nutrition, drugs—can give birth to a child who later develops mental health issues as they grow. Also, stressors such as divorce, low self-esteem, and loneliness can trigger a mental health condition.

2. Brain Chemistry

Brain chemicals, also known as neurotransmitters, transmit signals to all parts of the body and within the brain. If these chemicals are somehow impaired within the neural network, the nerve systems are affected. Mental disorders, such as depression and other mood dysregulation, could ensue. Several disorders have been linked to abnormal functioning of the nerve network and the pathways that connect the brain's various regions. Brain injuries and defects have also been linked to the development of certain mental illnesses because they disrupt these networks. Conditions such as epilepsy can also impact a person's mood and behavior.

3. Biological Factors

Genes play a huge part in mental illnesses. If one form of mental illness runs in a person's family, there's a huge possibility that one of their offspring could develop it. Sometimes, it isn't just because it runs in the family that increases the chances of developing it. An unfavorable situation, such as the loss of someone or financial problems, can trigger it without you even realizing. You only notice the abnormality when it becomes a regular occurrence.

However, experts have realized that even though a mental illness runs in the family, it's still possible to not inherit it. Susceptibility is passed from parents to their offspring through genes, but whether that mental illness develops depends on how the child interacts with their environment. Their temperament, upbringing, and life experiences also play a role.

How genes interact with the environment differs individually, and that's why two individuals from the same family may inherit the same susceptibility, but one of them will not develop the illness, while the other one will. Things like stress, abuse, or a traumatic event can trigger the manifestation of a mental illness in a person who has inherited susceptibility.

Infections can also trigger the development of mental illnesses, such as obsessive-compulsive behavior (OCD). For example, pediatric auto-immune neuropsychiatric disorder has been linked to OCD, especially in children.

Alcohol, drugs, and the Western diet are also known causes of mental health issues. Although research on the effects of diet and nutrition on mental health is still ongoing, so far, many researchers have established a relationship between Western diet—all our processed foods and abundance of sugars—and mental disorders. According to them, this diet can cause anxiety disorders and major depressive disorder.

The hippocampus area of the brain—responsible for the generation of new neurons—is linked to a person's mood and cognitive processes. One factor that can affect neurogenesis in adults and increase the risk of depression is a high fat and sugar diet. This explains why junk foods affect a person's mood.

4. Psychological Factors

Psychological factors include traumas (the loss of a parent or child), neglect as a child, sexual/physical/emotional abuse, etc. If you ever fought in combat as a soldier, the events that transpired during that period can trigger a mental illness, just like what happened to me after my deployment in Afghanistan.

In the course of my recovery from PTSD, my wife shared some great news with me—we were pregnant with our first son. That was indeed great, coming at a time when my recovery from PTSD was going smoothly and rapidly. It got more interesting when the church I always volunteered for ordained me as a deacon. It was all so perfect! During my one year of leadership training, my wife called me while I was at work and told me that my son had passed away. I rushed to the hospital and had to watch my wife give birth to a son that was no longer alive. It was unspeakably painful. But I had to be strong for her, like Superman. It was not easy. My PTSD reared its ugly head again—the loss of my son triggered it.

5. Social and Economic Factors

Social and economic pressure can cause the development of mental disorders. Changing jobs, losing a job, being poor/having limited finances, and belonging to a marginalized class can all cause and exacerbate mental health issues.

Shaming an individual because of their body size can also trigger mental illness. This is common amongst girls, and on more than one occasion, has led to the death of some individuals, many through suicide or substance abuse.

6. Mental Illness Triggers

Triggers are anything that can cause a person to remember a bad or traumatic experience. They can affect one's emotional state and leave the person overwhelmed with distress. Triggers affect an individual's ability to focus on the present and can influence their behavior. Sometimes, these triggers are also the causative factors of mental disorders. For example, eating junk food regularly is both a trigger and a cause of eating disorders, such as a binge eating disorder.

So, what are some examples of these triggers? Triggers are commonly divided into anxiety and trauma. In the list below, you will find triggers that are associated with anxiety and traumas. There are several of them, but I'll mention a few common ones.

- Seeing a picture or something that reminds you of someone close to you who died.

- Certain food types, especially junk and processed foods.
- If someone makes you angry or they are angry with you.
- The smell of alcohol and drugs.
- The smell of rotten food.
- As a former soldier, seeing soldiers on TV, military weapons, or several dead bodies on the ground.
- Political statements.
- Bodily waste, such as feces.
- Blood.
- A TV ad.
- Animals and insects.
- News updates.
- Anniversary dates, including birthday reminders.
- Loneliness.
- Being yelled at.
- Noises.
- Financial problems.
- Trying something new.
- Stress.
- Going out in public.
- Hearing words that were said during the traumatic event.

One of the best ways to fend off triggers is by surrounding yourself with positive people and understanding where they are coming from. When you surround yourself with the right people and individuals who each have mindsets focused on development, you can avoid triggers. Another great solution is to stay busy and motivated. Create a list of things to do, and make a habit of doing them, even if it takes you a significant amount of time. I will discuss other fantastic solutions in section four of this book.

Section Three:

PERCEPTION

Not everyone sees mental health problems the same way. Your perception of a situation will impact your mental health. Try to see things positively. It goes a long way. Dr. Courtney Miller has a video on YouTube titled *Mental Health Minute: The Power of Perception*. This video provides some insight on what exactly perception is when it comes to mental illness. Some have a negative perception of it, and as a result will often stigmatize those who they believe are suffering from a mental illness. Although public attitudes and behavior towards mental illnesses are improving, thanks to various awareness programs being staged all over the world, the stigma is still apparent. This stigma has been passed down to the younger generation, especially amongst men. However, as they tend to grow older, their understanding of the situation becomes clearer.

Mental illness is arguably the most common type of illness in the United States. According to the National Institute of Mental Health's survey, around 44.7 million adults in the United States suffered from a mental illness in 2016, and 43.1% of those received mental health services that year. These people comprised mostly Caucasian Americans, with African Americans, Hispanic Americans and Asian Americans receiving not more than one-third of mental health services. In 2006, mental health care-related expenditures ranked third in the costliest medical conditions.

In 2007, about 25% of adults with mental health disorders believed others were sympathetic towards patients with a mental illness. Perception and understanding of mental health have also improved in the United States, with institutions, relevant bodies, and even the media helping everyone realize that mental health issues are prevalent, and patients shouldn't be stigmatized. Still, an unbelievable number of people out there still discriminate against people with mental illness.

More than half of people with a mental disorder don't receive help due to concerns about being treated differently. These people fear that by being diagnosed with a mental health issue, they will lose their job and livelihood. This thought is so prevalent because the stigma and prejudice against people suffering from mental health issues stubbornly remains in existence. Stigma can be subtle or apparent, but none of it is justifiable. Discrimination can harm people. People with mental illness feel marginalized in so many ways. Therefore, understanding what it is will help in addressing it.

Stigma and Discrimination: The Bane of Untreated Mental Illnesses

Stigma is often blamed for untreated mental health conditions, but it comes from a lack of understanding of mental illnesses. The people who stigmatize have not been mentally ill themselves or have not personally known anyone with a mental health disorder. As a result, they don't understand the plight of those who are suffering. Inaccurate and misleading information from the media contributes to this. Studies on stigma reveal that, while the public accept the medical and genetic nature of a mental health disorder and the need for treatment, many still have a negative perception of mental illness.

According to the American Psychiatric Association, stigma is divided into three types—public, self, and institutional stigma. Public stigma is the discriminatory perception that others have about mental illness. This type of stigma labels people with mental illness as dangerous and incompetent. Self-stigma refers to the negative attitudes the patients cultivate towards themselves. They have internalized shame about their mental health conditions. These attitudes and thoughts result in low self-esteem. They question themselves, wondering if they are good enough or worthy of doing certain things, like being in specific positions, such as the head of an organization. Institutional stigma is systemic. It involves government policies and private laws that intentionally limit opportunities for people suffering from mental health issues. Examples of these policies include fewer mental health services and lower funding for research on mental illnesses.

Stigma affects not only the patients, it also affects their loved ones, family members, and friends. Those who support them are often discriminated against. The stigma of mental illness isn't unique to one country. It is universal. A 2016 study on stigma revealed that people with mental illnesses do not have the same societal value as those without them.

Effects of Stigmatization

Stigmatization can lead to worsening symptoms of mental illnesses and reduce the chances of getting treatment early or at all. Research reveals that those with self-stigma have a lower recovery rate among those diagnosed with mental disorders. Stigmatization and discrimination can reduce hope, lower self-esteem, affect social relationships, increase mental health symptoms, reduce chances of getting treatment, and decrease productivity at work.

Other harmful effects of stigma are a reluctance to seek help, isolation, fewer work opportunities, harassment and bullying, and negative beliefs that one won't ever succeed. Stigma is also a contributing factor when it comes to charitable fundraising to increase the availability of mental health services.

How to Fight Stigmatization and Adopt a Positive Perception

One of the best ways to reduce stigmatization is to have contact with someone who has dealt with mental health issues. By sharing their stories, these individuals can have a positive impact on society. When a celebrity that has battled mental illness speaks out about their journey, it becomes relatable and less scary. Celebrities like Demi Lovato, Dwayne "The Rock" Johnson, Taraji P. Henson, and Lady Gaga have publicly shared their mental health stories. Young people can learn from these examples, equip themselves with vital information, and learn that it is okay to talk about mental health.

Another effective strategy is engaging in social marketing campaigns. A research study revealed that an anti-stigma social media marketing campaign in California increased mental health services in the state by helping people understand what mental health illnesses entail. Other solutions to help reduce stigma include talking openly about it on social media, and educating yourself and others who have a shallow understanding of what mental health conditions are.

As an employer, you could encourage your workers to be open about their mental health struggles. Set up a program to monitor and offer support to those showing symptoms. Sponsor their treatments and make them aware that you care about their health, not just their work output. As an organization, start campaigns against stigmatization and discrimination. There are a couple of those out there, such as Make It Ok and Stamp Out Stigma.

You can change the negative perception of mental health illnesses. It starts with one voice, and another joins in, and eventually we can all rise up against stigmatization and discrimination.

Lastly, changing your own perception of your personal triggers and mental illness can go a long way. You may now view the world through eyes filtered by your hurt, trauma, triggers, and mental illness. So, be kind to yourself, because only you have your unique perception of what's going on. After COVID, the world became aware of the prevalence of some form of mental health trauma.

Section Four:

SUPPORT

As I explained in Section Two, coming home from Afghanistan left me riddled with pain. Unfortunately, I received no support from the military back home. At that time, I told my unit what was going on; that I was having nightmares and trouble sleeping. They simply told me to take some time off… but I knew that wouldn't help me, and that the unit wasn't ready to render the kind of support I truly needed.

Everyone treated me like I'd just returned from a vacation on one of those beautiful islands in Greece or the Maldives. There was no consideration for how I felt after the war. No one from the unit asked me what was going through my mind, whether or not I was living with trauma. Of course I felt traumatized. That's what war leaves you with.

So, I opted for a post-deployment assessment, because I knew it would help. It's a platform where you can share your experience or any issues you might be having. I put out a statement detailing my war experience to serve as a red flag that something was indeed going on with me, and hoping someone would reach out to me. Luckily, I got a call from a doctor who later helped me with my PTSD recovery. I was completely freed from the traumatic events that were impacting my productivity.

With the right support, you won't be reliving those hurtful moments when you saw your colleague get shot in the head or blasted to pieces by bombs. I'm not saying it will be easy, though. Having the courage to live through the pain can be one of the hardest things you'll ever do.

The effects of war, the death of your spouse, the breakdown of a marriage, losing a parent or child, are all things that can leave you incapacitated, and you may find it hard to inhibit the thoughts of suicide. With all that going on in your head, life happening around you may seem like too much for you to handle, and so you may feel like ending it all.

It's okay to feel this way. You are not alone.

It's a fact that only half of those who have mental health issues receive treatment, but that is not because there isn't help available to them. It is because of the stigma associated with getting that help, and the lack of understanding or knowledge of exactly what help is out there. The main causes of this stigma are media stereotypes and lack of education, and this tends to alter people's attitudes towards treating mental illness. Untreated mental issues can contribute to higher medical costs, poorer performance at your workplace or school, and a higher risk of committing suicide.

However, the good news is that there are still ways to get help if you have any sort of mental health issue. You can start by reaching out to your family members or friends. They will help you better understand why you need treatment, even if they do not fully understand what it is like living with a mental illness themselves. They will also be able to give you advice on where to go next and help you talk about what kind of treatment options are available in your area.

Perhaps talking with friends or family isn't enough. You still have other options. If that's the case, then contact your doctor or therapist immediately so they can refer you over to someone else who specializes in treating your specific issues.

As we've covered already, stigma is a *huge* problem in the mental health community. It affects everything from the availability of resources for treatment, to how people feel about reaching out to get that help. If you're struggling with mental health issues, it can be hard to find someone who will listen non-judgmentally and help you. In order to get treatment, we must make sure that stigma doesn't stand in the way.

First off, it's important to remember that, even if it may not feel like it, there's no shame in seeking help for your mental health. You are just as normal as anyone else. If someone tells you otherwise, don't listen to them. They're wrong! You deserve respect and acceptance, just like everyone else does.

If you feel accepted by others, chances are much higher that you'll get help because it will be easier for you to ask for what you need. Some ways you can show acceptance are by being open-minded when talking to other people about their struggles with mental health, asking questions instead of making assumptions, and not judging others based on their actions or appearances alone. Always remember that everyone deserves respect!

Having a strong support network is also vital when struggling with mental health issues. That could consist of support groups, family, or friends—you just need to have people who will listen without judgment as it can make all the difference between success or failure in your recovery.

Psychotherapy

One of the most popular means of treatment for mental health is psychotherapy. This chapter will discuss psychotherapy—its benefits, formats, types, and the tips necessary for making the most of it. Also, we will discuss other forms of mental health treatment.

The word psychotherapy comes from the Greek words "*psyche*" and "*therapeia*." These two words combined mean "breath and healing." Therefore, psychotherapy is a word that describes the treatment of disorders of the mind through psychological techniques.

In the past, psychotherapy was seen as the treatment of diseases through hypnosis. Psychotherapy is popularly called "talk therapy", however, many types of psychotherapy do not involve verbal communication. For this reason, the American Psychological Association agreed on a new definition of psychotherapy. The association's leaders defined psychotherapy as the application of clinical methods and interpersonal techniques derived from established psychological principles to help people modify their character, cognitions, emotions, and other personal behavior in the way they desire. The clinical methods used in the treatment are both intentional and informed.

Psychotherapy treatment helps in addressing spirituality as an essential part of an individual's mental state. Some formats came from spiritual philosophies, however, treatments based on spirituality are not considered conventional forms of psychotherapy.

Psychotherapy can be delivered in person, through the phone, or online. Also, you can attend a therapy session as an individual, a couple, or as part of a group. The modern development in psychotherapy has seen the use of computer-assisted therapy for behavioral exposure, with multimedia programs being created which can deliver various cognitive techniques.

Psychotherapy is internationally recognized as a form of mental illness treatment, but with slight variations in its delivery across the world. The process works for both adults and children.

Benefits of Psychotherapy

Many people who have been treated for mental illness see psychotherapy as a quintessential treatment because:

It helps overcome depression

Depression has many triggers, but the major cause is not yet known. Those suffering from depression can get help from their therapist. The therapist will help them recognize the triggers of their illness and train their mind in new ways that will help them respond better to those triggers.

Psychotherapy has been a significant means of treatment in mental health disorders. It has helped many people to get better at coping with depression and to do so without using medication. A study put together by the University of California in 2019 showed that people who used therapy to treat depression had a higher success rate than those who made use of prescription medication. It seems the study also shows that therapy is just as efficacious as medication, but more enduring.

Also, the former had less chance of relapsing into depression than the latter in the long term. Why is that?

It helps build more meaningful relationships

People with mental illness frequently live in isolation, and this is often because of the public stigma. Isolation leads to a worsening of anxiety, depression, and other cognitive problems in most cases. Therefore, it is difficult for such people to build and maintain healthy relationships with friends, colleagues, family members, or spouses.

It is easy to see why these people struggle with relationships when you consider how they are internally dysfunctional, which makes it difficult for them to relate to other people. Psychotherapy enables these people to recognize and correct the part of themselves that is dysfunctional. Therefore, they can build and maintain external relationships, as well as fix broken relationships.

It creates higher levels of peace and happiness

People with mental illness often have an overwhelming feeling of negativity buzzing through their minds. Finding relief from these negative thoughts for the first time can spur an exhilarating feeling of happiness and relief. As patients discover more ways to point out and defy these negative thoughts using healthy means, what started as preliminary relief can become a greater feeling of calmness and happiness in the long term.

It helps build confidence

Many people have one or two forms of personal insecurity they are dealing with. Those with psychological issues have a lower chance of possessing a decent level of self-confidence than others. But, talking to a mental health professional, and working with them as you confront your insecurities will make things a lot better. You will find small victories along the way, and most patients describe gaining a new sense of confidence, personally and professionally.

It helps to overcome anxiety

Anxiety is among the fastest-growing illnesses in the United States, as of 2023. From a survey carried out by the American Psychiatric

Association, a significant five percent increase in the national anxiety record in the country was identified. It also showed that more Americans are anxious now than in 2021.

About 20% of people suffering from anxiety sought professional help. Psychotherapy can assist patients in understanding their feelings and triggers. They can then learn to build better relationships with these feelings, which will make anxiety less likely to dominate their existence on a daily basis. Visiting a therapist that specializes in anxiety disorders can help patients observe the cause of their anxiety and create practical strategies to overcome them.

Formats of Psychotherapy

There are many formats of psychotherapy. The format used depends on the therapist. Also, the history and needs of the patient are deciding factors. Popular formats of psychotherapy include:

Individual therapy

This psychotherapy format involves working one-on-one with the therapist. Often, this method is used to help individuals overcome personal problems such as anxiety, depression, and low self-esteem.

Couples therapy

This form of therapy is used by therapists to address issues couples have in their relationship, such as communication and conflict resolution, and aims to help them overcome them.

Family therapy

The focus here is on family relationships. The format centers on making the dynamic within families more harmonious and positive and may involve multiple members within the family unit.

Group therapy

Here, the therapist works with a small group of individuals who all have similar goals. This format enables members of the group to provide and receive support from other group members, and then practice new behaviors within a supportive and receptive group environment.

Types of Psychotherapy

Most people think of psychotherapy as simply talking to a therapist. These people imagine a patient sitting or lying on a couch, while the therapist takes notes. However, psychotherapy involves more than that. Many techniques and practices are employed in psychotherapy. The method utilized in each therapy session depends on a variety of factors. Some of these factors include the training and background of the therapist, the choice of the client, and the nature of the client's mental illness.

Some of the popular types of psychotherapy include:

Cognitive-behavioral Therapy (CBT)

This type of therapy is one of the most prominent and is backed by a lot of evidence proving its efficacy. Commonly referred to as CBT, this type of therapy helps patients recognize the thoughts and emotions that influence their behavior. CBT treats a variety of conditions, such as phobias, addiction, depression, and anxiety.

CBT deploys cognitive and behavioral strategies to alter negative thoughts. The method assists people suffering from mental illness to change underlying thoughts that bring distress and amend problematic responses to triggers.

Humanistic Therapy

This type of therapy began in the 1950s with the school of thought called "humanistic psychology." Carl Rogers established an approach called client-centered therapy, which concentrated on the therapist showing thorough and unconditional positive regard to the client. Aspects of this method are still used today. The humanistic method of psychotherapy concentrates on helping people maximize their potential and stresses the validity of self-exploration, free will, and self-actualization.

Cognitive Therapy

The cognitive revolution of the 1960s had a significant impact on the practice of psychotherapy. Cognitive psychologists focused more on how human thought processes affect behavior and functioning. For example, if you often see negativity in every circumstance, you will probably have a pessimistic outlook and a gloomier overall mood. The purpose of cognitive therapy is to spot the cognitive biases that create negative thoughts and replace them with more optimistic and realistic ones. Through this means, people suffering from mental illness can improve their moods and overall well-being.

Psychoanalysis

Although psychotherapy existed in many forms, going back to ancient Greece, formal recognition of the practice only started when Sigmund Freud began using the method to work with patients. Techniques often employed by Freud were the analysis of transference, dream interpretation, and free association.

The crucial thing about this approach is the need to delve into an individual's thoughts and previous life experiences to identify unconscious thoughts, emotions, and memories that impact their character and behavior.

Eye Movement Desensitization Reprocessing Therapy (EMDR)

EMDR is another form of psychotherapy that is used to treat anxiety disorders like PTSD. It is similar to exposure therapy in the sense that it alleviates the emotional distress sustained from traumatic events. A mindfulness technique is used in the following way: A patient pays attention to sounds and movements while reminiscing on their traumatic memories. EMDR stimulation is then done until those memories become less distressing. A few sessions of EMDR can be enough to relieve you of symptoms of PTSD, but in severe cases, 1-3 months of 90-minute weekly sessions are required for the best results.

Acceptance and Commitment Therapy (ACT)

ACT is a psychotherapeutic technique that teaches patients to always remain positive in the face of adversity. It encourages patients to engage in positive behaviors instead of negative behaviors.

Let's say a person is struggling with social anxiety and tends to avoid social situations. They have a strong desire to make friends and be more socially active, but their fear and self-doubt prevent them from taking action. In an ACT session, the therapist might use the following approach:

- Acceptance: The therapist helps the individual recognize and accept their anxious thoughts and feelings. Instead of trying to suppress or eliminate these emotions, the person acknowledges them as a natural part of their experience.

- Diffusion: The therapist assists the individual in distancing themselves from their anxious thoughts. They might use techniques such as thought labeling or metaphors to help the person see their thoughts as just thoughts, rather than as objective truths or barriers to action.

- Clarifying Values: The therapist helps the person identify their core values regarding social connections and meaningful relationships. They explore what kind of person the individual wants to be in the context of social interactions.

- Commitment to Action: The therapist encourages the person to take small, manageable steps towards their values-based goals. This might involve attending a social event, starting a conversation with someone new, or joining a social club.

- Mindfulness: The therapist guides the individual in practicing mindfulness techniques to stay present and nonjudgmental during social interactions. This helps them to observe their anxious thoughts and feelings without being overwhelmed by them, allowing for more intentional and value-driven behavior.

ACT doesn't solely focus on being positive, but rather on accepting and working with difficult thoughts and emotions while taking meaningful action aligned with personal values. By using ACT techniques, individuals can learn to engage in positive behaviors despite adversity or uncomfortable internal experiences.

This treatment is effective for patients suffering from generalized anxiety disorder (GAD) and depression, especially in cases of those disorders that are highly resistant. The length of treatment varies and depends on the severity of symptoms.

Dialectical Behavioral Therapy (DBT)

DBT is a skill-based technique that is effective in the treatment of personality and anxiety disorders, as well as PTSD. DBT focuses on developing skills, and how patients can use those developed skills to manage stress, regulate their emotions, and improve interpersonal relationships. This therapy takes time, usually over a year, to achieve the desired results, but most patients who undergo this therapy recover and get better.

Prolonged Exposure Therapy

Prolonged exposure therapy is specifically designed to treat PTSD and phobias. In confronting fears, the patient can overcome the distress they feel about trauma-related experiences. During exposure therapy, the therapist employs a careful method to introduce memories to the patient. The therapist then guides the patient into using coping techniques, such as relaxation therapy, to deal with those traumas. The therapist reminds the patient that those traumatic experiences or memories are in the past and pose no current threats to them. Eight to 16 weeks is the expected duration of this therapy.

Where Psychotherapy Can Help

Although many types of psychotherapy exist, they all serve the same purpose—helping people overcome challenges, create coping techniques, and enabling them to enjoy happier and healthy lives. People experiencing symptoms of psychological or psychiatric disorders can benefit from evaluation by a certified and experienced psychotherapist who can assess, diagnose, and treat mental illness.

Psychotherapy is effective in treating many mental health issues, including:

- Addiction
- All forms of anxiety disorders
- Depression
- Eating disorders
- Post-traumatic stress disorder
- Substance abuse
- Bipolar disorder
- Obsessive-compulsive disorder
- Chronic pain
- Break-ups
- Grief
- Sleep disorders
- Low self-confidence
- Stress

How to Maximize Psychotherapy Sessions

The effectiveness of therapy depends on many factors. First, the nature and stringency of the problem. Second, your willingness to maximize your time. Below are ways you can make the most of your sessions:

Be honest with your therapist

If you withhold your emotions from the therapist, they can't help you overcome your problems. The goal is to show up as your true and authentic self, without attempting to conceal any part of your personality that you are afraid to let others see.

Be open to the process

You must work to establish an open and real therapeutic alliance with your therapist. Some surveys reveal that therapy works best when you feel a genuine connection with the therapist treating you.

Attend your session consistently

Life happens… and sometimes you are too busy to attend sessions. However, you have to make a conscious effort to follow your treatment plan and schedule appointments that enable you to consistently attend sessions.

Express your feelings

It is best to express any negative feeling such as grief, anger, anxiety, or fear during a therapy session. The purpose of therapy is to talk about these feelings in a safe space. So, if you hide them, you defeat the purpose.

Do the work

When you are assigned a task to complete at home by your therapist, it is best to do it before your next appointment. If you can complete all your assignments on time, it will make the healing process more efficient.

Things to Consider Before Starting Therapy

There are many things to consider for both the therapist and the patient. When rendering services to patients, psychotherapists should consider issues like informed consent, patient confidentiality, and their responsibility to warn authorities of the patient's risk to themselves or others.

Informed consent means acquainting the patient with all the inherent risks and advantages that treatment involves. For example, the therapist should explain the real nature of the treatment, the risks and costs associated with it, and the alternatives available to the patient.

Therapists also have a duty to warn, which means explaining that, as a therapist, they are legally required to inform the authorities if a client intends to cause harm to themselves or others. It is one of the few exceptions where therapist-client confidentiality can be breached. Apart from that, since clients talk about issues that are so deeply personal and sensitive, psychotherapists have a legal obligation to protect their client's right to confidentiality.

How to Start Therapy

Psychotherapy is an effective treatment for many psychological challenges, and like regularly seeing a doctor, it is best to seek help before you become overwhelmed by the symptoms of your mental illness. The sooner you seek help, the quicker you will be able to live a healthier, more peaceful life.

It is best to consider the following before going to your first therapy session:

Talk to your primary care physician

Your doctor may rule out any physical disease that is responsible for your symptoms. If they can't find any physical cause, you may be referred to a mental health professional trained to diagnose and treat mental illness.

Search for a qualified individual

Those who provide psychotherapy may have several titles or degrees. For example, they can be a psychologist or psychiatrist or social worker. These fields all have special licensing requirements.

Individuals certified to offer psychotherapy services include licensed counselors, licensed social workers, psychologists, psychiatrists, and advanced nurse practitioners.

Addressing Substance Use Disorder Before Treating Mental Illness

1. Substance use can mimic or exacerbate the symptoms of mental illness, making it difficult to establish an accurate diagnosis. Treating SUD as a priority allows for a clearer understanding of the underlying mental health condition.

2. Stabilization: Addiction can be all-consuming, and it may be challenging for individuals to fully engage in therapy for

mental illness while actively using substances. Achieving sobriety provides a stable foundation for addressing mental health concerns.

3. Enhanced Treatment Efficacy: Addressing SUD first can increase the effectiveness of subsequent mental health treatment. With drugs or alcohol no longer clouding judgment or numbing emotions, therapy and medication can better target the root causes of the mental health condition.

4. Reduced Relapse Risk: Attempting to treat mental illness without addressing addiction may lead to frequent relapses. By breaking the cycle of substance abuse, individuals can build resilience against relapse and focus on lasting recovery.

The Importance of Integrated Treatment

Integrated treatment models, which address both SUD and mental health issues simultaneously, have gained recognition as an effective approach. This approach acknowledges the interconnected nature of these conditions and provides a comprehensive treatment plan that includes therapy, counseling, medical intervention, and support services.

Seeking Help: The First Step Towards Recovery

- Reaching out for help is the crucial first step for individuals caught in the web of SUD and mental illness. Its essential to connect with healthcare professionals who can assess the severity of both conditions and tailor a treatment plan accordingly. This plan may involve detoxification, rehabilitation, therapy, medication, and ongoing support to achieve and maintain sobriety.

- It's important for individuals to remember that recovery is a unique journey, and there is no one-size-fits-all solution. Patience, commitment, and a strong support system are vital components of the recovery process.

- Addressing substance use disorder before embarking on therapy for mental illness is often a necessary and prudent approach. By prioritizing sobriety, individuals can gain better control over their mental health, leading to a more hopeful and sustainable path towards overall well-being and recovery.

Select the right therapist

When choosing a therapist, it is crucial to choose someone you feel most comfortable with, because it will be easier to talk to them about your deepest feelings and issues. In addition, it is important to consider the qualification of the therapist, alongside their years of experience. Referrals from friends and family members are a good place to start when searching for a therapist, as well as a referral from your preferred family medical practitioner.

Don't hesitate to consult different therapists

If you don't notice any change after a few sessions with the therapist you chose, it's okay to try another one! In fact, it is best to continue looking until you get one that you really connect with and with whom you feel comfortable.

Alternative Treatments for Mental Health Illnesses

There are other methods of treating mental illness besides psychotherapy. We will look at some of them below:

Case Management

Case management is a strategy that originated in the United States in response to the closure of state psychiatric hospitals. Initially, it aimed to provide services previously offered by these now-closed institutions. Over time, it evolved to include clinical or therapeutic case management as the need for mental health professionals to establish therapeutic relationships grew. One notable approach is assertive community treatment, which takes a holistic and integrated approach to psychiatric case management, enhancing wellness for the individuals it serves.

The functions of case management encompass various aspects:

1. Outreach and patient identification.
2. Service or care planning.
3. Review of individual needs.
4. Plan implementation.
5. Progress monitoring.
6. Continuous review and program termination.

When a reassessment identifies multiple needs that require systemic interventions, a new case management cycle begins. Case managers play a pivotal role in understanding the social system, identifying client needs, and ensuring effective service delivery while maintaining patient records. Modern record-keeping often employs checklists and scan sheets for statistical management.

In essence, case management serves as a vital link between patients and their care delivery system, adapting to evolving needs and focusing on improving the well-being of those it serves.

Models of Case Management

Many models of case management exist to coordinate care for people with diverse needs and for whom re-assessment is required. Typically, outcome evaluations determine the effectiveness of treatment interventions. Therefore, researchers have established fidelity measures to evaluate the progress of specific case management models. Below are some popular examples of case management models:

Clinical case management

This model requires the involvement of a case manager in the treatment process, with a one-on-one case manager-to-client relationship.

Assertive community treatment

The focus of this model is reduced hospital time. A multidisciplinary team comprising 10 or 12 members works as case managers, but the client remains one person.

Brokerage model

In this model, the aim is to connect clients to services. A single case manager is needed who will attend to one individual.

Personal empowerment model

Alternatively, this model is called the "strengths model" and was developed in the 1980s. The focus of the model is on the abilities and interests of the client. One case manager is used, and they engage one individual. The effectiveness of the model is measured with a strengths model fidelity scale.

Team case management

Here, the focus varies to suit the needs of the client. A team of case managers is needed with this model. Nonetheless, the client remains an individual. There is no fidelity scale to measure the effectiveness of the model. Under this model, a group of clients is catered to simultaneously.

Cluster case management

This model year of development is unknown. However, it provides multiple supports as it's a central focus. A single case manager is used, but sometimes assistants are employed.

Intensive case management

The purpose of this model is to reduce hospital and emergency service use. One case manager is used under this model, and a single person is treated at a time. A systematic review investigates the impact of intensive case management on clients with serious mental illness.

Natural Remedies

There are also natural remedies that can curb the symptoms of anxiety and other mental illnesses. The good thing about these lifestyle changes is that you can use them along with medication and psychological treatments. Lifestyle changes include:

Limiting Caffeine and Alcohol Consumption

Caffeine is not bad, but it may trigger higher levels of anxiety when consumed excessively. The same goes for alcohol. Sometimes, we may feel that turning to alcohol is the best way to manage the anxiety brought on by our busy work schedules and other engagements, but it is not. On the contrary, we will be weakening our liver and our body and making things worse.

According to the Department of Agriculture's Dietary Guidelines for Americans, the recommended amount of caffeine for adults is 400 mg per day. That is the amount found in two to four eight-ounce cups of coffee. Anything more than that is unhealthy. The same guidelines recommend drinking alcohol moderately, which means one drink per day for women and two for men.

Avoid Junk Foods and Eat a Balanced Diet

As comforting as they can be, junk foods will cause you more harm than good. Junk foods are tied to obesity, which can negatively impact your heart rate and can lead to heart disease and other diseases like diabetes. Eating a balanced, healthy diet will calm your anxiety levels and help regulate your body's systems. I recommend foods like fatty fish, eggs, dark chocolate, turmeric, yogurt, and pumpkin seeds. Fruits like citrus and strawberries can also help fight stress and ease anxiety levels.

1. Fatty Fish (Salmon, Mackerel, Trout): Fatty fish are rich in omega-3 fatty acids, particularly EPA and DHA. These nutrients are known for their anti-inflammatory properties, which can

help reduce inflammation in the brain and potentially alleviate symptoms of anxiety and depression. Additionally, omega-3s support overall brain health and function.

2. Eggs: Eggs are a source of several nutrients that play a role in mental health, including choline and vitamin D. Choline is a precursor to acetylcholine, a neurotransmitter that is essential for memory and mood regulation. Adequate vitamin D levels are associated with lower rates of depression and anxiety.

3. Dark Chocolate (in moderation): Dark chocolate contains compounds like flavonoids, which have antioxidant properties and can improve blood flow to the brain. It also contains a small amount of caffeine, which can boost alertness and mood. However, moderation is key, as excessive sugar content can have adverse effects.

4. Turmeric: Turmeric contains curcumin, a potent anti-inflammatory compound. Chronic inflammation has been linked to various mental health issues, including depression and anxiety. Curcumin's ability to reduce inflammation may contribute to its potential mood-lifting effects.

5. Yogurt (Probiotic-Rich Foods): Yogurt and other probiotic-rich foods support gut health. The gut-brain connection is a growing area of research, and a healthy gut microbiome is believed to influence mood and mental health positively. Probiotics can help maintain a balanced gut flora, which may indirectly benefit mental well-being.

6. Pumpkin Seeds: Pumpkin seeds are a good source of magnesium. Magnesium is essential for regulating neurotransmitters and has a calming effect on the nervous system. It may help reduce symptoms of anxiety and stress.

7. Citrus Fruits and Strawberries: These fruits are high in vitamin C, which is an antioxidant that can help combat oxidative stress in the body. Oxidative stress has been linked to mood disorders, so a diet rich in vitamin C can provide protection against this.

These foods are chosen for their potential to support mental health through various mechanisms. Some are anti-inflammatory, helping to reduce chronic inflammation that can contribute to mood disorders. Others support gut health, which is closely connected to the production of neurotransmitters like serotonin, often referred to as the "happy hormone." Incorporating a balanced diet that includes these foods can complement therapeutic interventions and promote overall well-being. However, its essential to remember that while diet plays a role, it should be part of a comprehensive approach to mental health, including professional guidance and self-care practices.

Getting Sufficient Sleep

Sometimes workdays can be so stressful and tiring that you have no time or energy left to take care of yourself. Life is all about balance—you need to find a way to balance your work and rest. Getting enough sleep helps relax the body and refresh the mind. This means that each time you wake up, the body feels revitalized, re-energized, and ready to kickstart or continue from where it left off.

Increasing Physical Activity

Exercise is a great way to burn calories. But did you know that exercising can also lessen anxiety? Yes, it's true, exercise can treat anxiety really effectively. It is also helpful for those who want to quit smoking. Relaxation exercises are also great for people with tense muscles. By relaxing the muscles, blood flows better, releasing the tension between the muscles. This then helps relax the entire body—including the mind.

Practicing Meditation and Mindfulness

Meditation and breathing exercises can help treat anxiety. Meditation and mindfulness can slow racing thoughts, calm the mind, and help with improving mood.

Journaling

Writing is the ultimate expression of what you feel, and getting your thoughts down on paper can be extremely therapeutic. By expressing your thoughts and feelings, you create a path to let go of what is causing you anxiety. Additionally, creative writing can help you manage anxiety by creating a distraction, making you focus on what you are putting down on paper rather than what's worrying you.

Build Your Support Network

Building a strong support network can help people cope with anxiety. Research has shown that having good social support reduces the symptoms of PTSD. Talking and connecting with a group of good friends can ease anxiety symptoms. You can take part in group activities, join social clubs, and lean on your family. You can also get involved in societal topics and issues affecting humanity, sports, and entertainment, too.

Aromatherapy

Aromatherapy can help you overcome headaches, depression, stress, and anxiety levels. Certain scents from soothing plant oils like lavender, eucalyptus, peppermint, chamomile, and bergamot help slow down our heart rate in the short term and ease insomnia in the long term. This might not work for everybody, but you should try it. If you do not want to inhale these scents, you can use the essential oils from these plants on your body. Mix or dilute them with your cream or body wash and apply them directly to your skin. Never apply essential oils directly to the skin.

Maintain Good Eating Habits

Eating late at night or close to when you go to sleep is unhealthy and will alter your body's systems. This will make your body work at digesting that food when it ought to be resting, thus raising your stress levels.

Support Groups

Another alternative means of treating mental illness is to engage in support groups. It doesn't matter if you are dealing with chronic illness, emotional issues, or want to improve your overall health, there will be a group within your community that is made up of people in the same situation! Let's look at how a support group can help you.

A support group is made of people in the same situation that may help you fill the void. In ancient times, square dances, quilting bees, and other community gatherings were common examples of places where many people came together to celebrate, encourage, and support one another. In modern times, most people need the same encouragement, consolation, and nurturing, especially during times of crisis. However, face-to-face interaction within the community is scarcer than ever. Those who are lucky receive support from family members and friends. Nevertheless, they may not always understand the intricacies of your situation.

For this reason, you need a support group of people in the same situation or circumstances as you. They will understand what you are going through. Support groups consist of regular meetings where people with similar problems come together to support and encourage each other. In the last few years, there has been an increase in the number of support groups for various disorders, illnesses, and challenges, and is something you should make the most of!

Forms of Support Groups Available

There are support groups for a variety of challenges. Below are common examples of support groups you can find in your neighborhood.

Chronic illnesses

People who are suffering from diseases such as cancer, post-traumatic stress disorder, depression, anxiety, or other mental health problems can share their experiences in these groups, and will help new members of the group learn their coping strategies.

Situational crisis groups

Members of these groups include the newly divorced, unemployed, single parents, widows or widowers, caregivers, and those living with life-threatening issues such as terminal illness.

Personal growth and wellness groups

These groups include people who want to lose weight, quit smoking, and exercise more. Often, members of these groups include both genders.

Family support group

Members of these groups include people that help members cope with the illnesses of their family members or loved ones.

What to Expect from a Support Group

There are a great variety of experiences when it comes to support groups, but all groups share one thing in common—they are the perfect place for people to share personal stories, express their feelings, and be heard in a space of acceptance, understanding, and encouragement.

Members use them as spaces to exchange information and resources. Through helping others, people belonging to a support group strengthen and empower themselves. Additionally, providing support helps some groups focus on community education.

Emotional support received from participation helps people reduce stress, which can affect their health positively. In addition, people can benefit from the information exchange that takes place in a support group by learning to manage symptoms, develop better coping skills, and communicate more openly with their therapists.

And the benefits extend beyond the person attending. Participation in support groups helps partners, friends, and family members also learn how to be more understanding and supportive of their loved ones who attend. Overall, the benefits received from support groups reduce stress and improve recovery outcomes considerably.

How to Locate a Support Group

Many communities have support groups of various kinds. If you are searching for a support group, then a community page in your phone book, on social media, in local newspapers, or online are all good places to start. You can also ask your caregiver or therapist for information about support groups.

But what if I have a problem that has no relevant group in my community? Well, then you might consider starting a support group.

You could let your doctor/therapist know about your plan to start a support group and give them your number to pass out so that others can join. Also, consider letting people know about the support group using community pages in your local newspaper, or distribute flyers to doctors, libraries, and parks.

Complementary and Alternative Medicine

Though they are not widely accepted, people suffering from mental illness can benefit from complementary and alternative therapies that are not part of traditional medical care. Alternative therapies, also known as complementary and alternative medicine (CAM) or integrative therapies, refer to a wide range of healthcare practices that are used in addition to or instead of conventional medical treatments. These therapies are considered alternative because they often differ from the conventional approaches used in Western medicine. Alternative therapies include acupuncture, herbal medicine, chiropractic care, homeopathy, naturopathy, Ayurveda, energy healing, and mind-body interventions.

Research has shown that complementary therapies can increase wellbeing, promote relaxation, and facilitate improved mental health. Also, alternative medicine is effective for different mental health needs and symptoms. Although the popularity of complementary medicine has increased in recent times, many people are not aware of its effectiveness yet.

What is Complementary and Alternative Medicine?

This type of medicine differs from traditional medical care. Therefore, you won't get this type of medical care from the hospital or your primary care doctor. You also shouldn't stop seeking care from those places, because alternative medicine is mostly only used as a complement to traditional treatment. However, in some cases, it can serve as an alternative to conventional medication.

Types of Complementary and Alternative Medicine

Here are common examples:

Acupuncture

This procedure is based on ancient Chinese practices. The procedure involves the use of small, thin needles that pierce the skin at certain points of the body. Practitioners believe these needles can assist the healing process in the body.

Using acupuncture for mental health treatment has become popular. There is ongoing research into its effectiveness in treating depression, insomnia, and schizophrenia. However, there is no scientific evidence supporting the claim that acupuncture is effective in treating mental illness at the moment.

Herbal solutions

Herbs can treat patients—sometimes referred to as herbal medicine—quite effectively, and if you are feeling skeptical, then it helps to keep in mind that most traditional drugs are manufactured from products originating from plants.

Herbs exist in a variety of forms, such as powders, teas, creams, and liquids. A certified herbalist may prescribe herbal concoctions to use as a complement to other medications or treatment methods. However, it is best to check if the herbal remedy is certified before buying it. The certification implies that medical trials have been carried out on the herbal remedy and positive results have been recorded from its use. Also, this shows that it is safe for consumption. However, it is best to talk to your doctor before starting any herbal remedy, because they can affect your health negatively, and there may be some interactions between herbal remedies and any prescription medication you are on. Some herbs I found that helped me are l-theanine and ashwagandha.

Massage

A massage therapist uses massage techniques to help eliminate tension and improve relaxation. There are many forms of massage, some of them are:

- Swedish massage – long kneading strokes, rhythmic, light tapping strokes, and movement of the joints to relax muscles and get rid of tension.
- Shiatsu massage – pressure is placed on certain points of the body to create a balance of energy.

Meditation

Meditation teaches you to maintain your focus on your mind and body. It is an excellent way to pay attention to the present moment. An example of mindfulness meditation would be focusing on your breathing. Consider how you feel after breathing in and out a few times.

Practicing meditation and mindfulness will make it easier to learn how to control your emotions. Also, it will be easier to deal with them. Mindfulness-based cognitive therapy (MBCT) is one of the most popular forms of mindfulness therapy available and is a combination of mindfulness meditation and cognitive-behavioral therapy (CBT).

A survey carried out by the healthcare profession revealed that

MBCT can help people overcome depression. MBCT courses typically last eight weeks are usually carried out in groups, with a session usually lasting around two hours. At the end of your therapy course, it is best to have a follow-up session a year later.

Alternatively, you can find mindfulness courses in self-help books or guides, mobile apps, podcasts, or by watching YouTube videos. You can also find classes in your local community.

Homeopathy

Homeopathy is based on the notion that the substance responsible for a symptom similar to the one produced by the ailment will also help reduce the symptom if used in minute doses. During this process, substances are diluted and shaken.

Practitioners of homeopathy believe that the substance will have more impact on symptoms if it is watered down significantly. However, the efficacy of homeopathy is still controversial.

Yoga

Yoga is a physical practice that focuses on learning breathing techniques, building strength, and increasing flexibility. Yoga helps people improve their mental and physical health. Physiotherapists have shown that yoga is effective in reducing depression, anxiety, and stress.

Yoga classes are available in your local gym and online. Also, there are yoga mobile apps that will help you get into it from the comfort of your own home.

Spiritual and energy healing

Spiritual healers believe that "energy" within the body impacts your mental and physical health. An example of one of these practices is Reiki. During this procedure, the therapist places their hands on specific areas of your body. Movement across these areas is believed to channel the energy of the body. For this reason, the therapist can direct energy flow to help the healing of the body and mind. During this procedure, you can keep your clothes on and either sit or lie down.

Although the effect of Reiki on mental health remains relatively unknown, it has shown some efficacy in reducing symptoms of depression, anxiety, stress, and sleep disorders.

How to Get Complementary and Alternative Therapies

You can receive complementary and alternative therapies through the following:

- Visiting a health spa for massages or acupuncture.
- Alternative therapy centers for homeopathy or Reiki.
- Hiring a private therapist or practitioners.
- Some mental health centers offer alternative therapies.

Things to Consider Before Choosing a Practitioner

Practitioners of complementary and alternative medicine don't need to become certified before they can attend to clients. However, it would be best to work with a practitioner that is part of a professional body, because they will have to adhere to a rigorous code of conduct. Also, they will stick to the ethics of their profession because they will not want to lose their license. It is essential to consider the following before selecting a practitioner:

- Compare the cost of therapies to ensure you don't overpay for services.

- Find out about the certification, and their membership in a professional body.
- Do your research and find testimonials from past clients.
- Select a practitioner that best meets your needs.
- Find out what to expect from the procedure. You want as much information as possible.
- Ask the practitioner how the treatment works, including any potential side effects.

Self-Care as a Treatment for Mental Illness

It is difficult to live with mental illness and can seem like a constant problem that has no visible solution. Although medication and psychotherapy are effective in alleviating the condition, some people suffering from mental illness need day-to-day monitoring to feel good, or even okay.

Exercise and meditation are common examples of self-help for people suffering from mental illness. These examples are helpful to a few people. However, other effective methods are not mentioned often enough. We will look at some of these simple techniques that you can include in your daily routine.

Radical acceptance

Radical acceptance describes a state of mind where you accept something completely, from deep within your heart and soul. An excellent example is to imagine a hurricane coming towards your city. Of course, you can't stop a hurricane. However, if you resign yourself to the fact that it is coming, then you can take steps to keep yourself safe. On the contrary, if you decide to will the hurricane away and do not prepare, then you will be in real danger when it hits!

The same scenario applies to mental illness. You can't do anything to change the fact that you have a mental illness. Therefore, don't spend your time trying to eliminate it by force of will or pretending you don't have it. Doing these things will only waste your time and energy.

Instead, accept yourself and the condition for what it is. Then, take the required steps necessary to manage the situation and take care of yourself.

Mental reframing

This process involves taking an emotion or trigger and changing the way you think about it. For example, instead of thinking how horrible your life is because of your mental illness, see it as a challenge you will overcome. Perfecting this method is tough, but it can make you feel better about any situation and is worth the time and practice required to get it right.

Deep breathing

Many people have spoken about how effective deep breathing is. It is one of the best ways to relieve stress and calm anxiety. Deep breathing helps you clear your head. It is best to think of it as a reset button.

You can try the following deep breathing technique:

- Breathe in for five seconds.
- Hold that breath for at least three seconds, and breathe out for seven seconds.

This easy repetition delivers a message of serenity to your brain and assures it that everything is fine or will soon be fine. After a short time, your heart will slow, and you will feel more relaxed.

Emotional understanding

If you continue to deny your emotions, it will be more difficult to take care of them. However, if you identify your emotions, you can tackle them or whatever is responsible for them. Therefore, if you are feeling stressed, go ahead and allow yourself to be stressed for a few minutes! Then meditate.

It is best to keep in touch with your emotions. Then accept what you feel before you act. Always remember that you can't control your mental illness, but you can decide how to respond to its symptoms.

Although this step is not easy, practice and perfecting the coping strategies can improve how you feel emotionally, spiritually, and mentally.

The five senses strategy

People with mental illness can turn to their physical space to ground themselves during a crisis. The technique is known as "the five senses." Rather than focusing on a particular subject with your five senses, run through each one of them individually and notice what they are experiencing at the moment. Running through all your five senses will require only a few seconds and will help you remain focused and grounded in the present. Also, it will help you separate reality from your imagination.

Things You Can Do to Improve Your Mental Health

An essential part of maintaining your mental health is taking care of your physical health. Staying healthy becomes even more important if you are currently suffering from mental illness. Since the symptoms of mental illness are difficult to overcome, you need to take your mental health seriously.

In this chapter, we will look at things you do to improve your mental health.

Maintain adequate sleep patterns

Sleep is essential to our physical and mental well-being. It helps regulate the hormones in our brain, which send information to other parts of the body. These hormones are responsible for our mood and emotions. Therefore, lack of adequate sleep disrupts the function of these hormones, which will negatively affect our mood. To improve your sleep patterns, do the following:

- Create a sleep-inducing bedroom environment.
- Establish a sleep schedule and stick to it.
- Create a pre-bedtime ritual.

Stay away from alcohol, drugs, and smoking

Drinking, drug-taking, and smoking can easily have a negative impact on our mental health. For example, after having a few drinks, you will probably feel more depressed the next day. It will be more difficult to concentrate on tasks. Heavy drinking over a long period can also cause thiamine deficiency, which is a hormone that is essential to brain function. Also, thiamine deficiency causes confusion, eye problems, feeling of nervousness, and coordination problems.

Smokers will become irritated and anxious between cigarettes. Taking illicit drugs, or abusing prescription medication, will cause mood swings and anxiety and only make things worse. In addition, drugs can add to symptoms of paranoia and delusions and may even result in overdose or death. Some psychiatrists believe excessive drug use can actually cause schizophrenia.

The following steps can help you quit smoking:

- Set up stop-smoking sessions.
- Understanding your smoking triggers and finding ways to avoid them.
- Stay busy and/or exercise to keep cravings at bay.
- Speak to a therapist about nicotine replacement therapy.
- Find ways to manage your stress better.

On the other hand, you can overcome alcohol and drug abuse problems by:

- Getting therapy.
- Attending inpatient or outpatient rehab.
- Changing your routine and environment. If you live close to a bar, it might be best to move! Also, if your colleagues often go to the bar after work, it would be best to change friends or departments to avoid that temptation to join. Or maybe explain the problem to a colleague you trust to avoid being invited.

For those with drug abuse problems, it is best to seek professional help to overcome them.

Spend time in the sun

Sunlight is an excellent source of vitamin D. It is called the "sunshine vitamin" and is crucial to our bodies and brains. Vitamin D helps release hormones in the brain that improve our mood. Perfect examples of these hormones are endorphins and serotonin. It is, therefore, best to go out in the sun as much as you can, but ensure you protect your skin and eyes. To get the required amount of vitamin D, spend at least 30 minutes, but not more than two hours, in the sun every day.

Manage stress

Let's face it, stress is not something you can eliminate from your life. However, if you know how to cope with it, your mental health won't be as affected. An excellent way to manage stress is to make a list of your responsibilities and worries and create a plan for resolving each issue.

Most times, if you write down your worries and stresses, you will find it easier to manage them. Try not to think about all your problems at once. If the stress is affecting your sleep, write all those worries down, then consciously decide to handle them later.

Engage in activities you enjoy

It is essential to do things you enjoy. For example, going for a walk, painting, playing a sport, or watching your favorite TV shows are some activities you could get absorbed in to help you manage stress. Research has shown that doing what you love improves your mood and makes you happy.

If you don't know what you enjoy doing, talk to your friends or colleagues about planning an activity.

Stay active and exercise

Exercise is vital in maintaining good mental health. Staying active not only gives you a sense of accomplishment, but also enhances self-confidence and improves your mood. Also, exercise boosts the hormones in your brain that help put you in a positive mood. Regular exercise can help you manage anxiety, stress, bad moods, and will even boost your life expectancy. You don't have to take part in a marathon or play basketball for four quarters every day! A short walk or light jog once a day is enough.

Help others

Helping people benefits both you and the person you are helping. Helping someone can improve your self-esteem and make you feel good about yourself. It makes you feel like you belong to the community and are needed. Volunteering for a local charity or being a good neighbor are great ways to start. You don't have to spend all your time helping people or volunteering, just spending a week at a local charity or doing community service on Saturday mornings is sufficient.

Seek help

We spoke about this in the previous chapter, but we shall discuss it more in this chapter. One of the best ways to stay on top of your mental health is to identify when you need help. You don't have to be ashamed of asking someone for support if you are anxious or stressed. Also, remember that no one is entirely free from stress. If you have suicidal thoughts or ideation, you should tell someone close to you and contact a suicide helpline immediately. Speak to your friends or family they can help. However, if you feel you might be suffering from a mental illness, speak to your doctor immediately.

Connect with others and become sociable

Try to establish and maintain a good rapport with people around you. Also, connect with friends and loved ones and make time for the people you care about. Having friends is crucial to feeling supported and receiving help when you need it. Research by mental health experts shows that talking to others can also boost memory and boost productivity.

Eat a balanced diet

Eating well is crucial to the development of our bodies and minds. Deficiencies in minerals such as iron and vitamin B12 can have a devastating effect on mental and physical health. So, it is essential to eat a balanced diet, especially if you are constantly stressed or anxious, or have been diagnosed with a mental illness.

Keep track of gratitude and accomplishments with a diary

This exercise is a simple way to relieve stress. Start by getting a journal. At the end of each day, write down three things you are grateful for, and three things you achieved that day.

If you do this consistently, you will feel better about your days. This exercise will help you see your accomplishments clearly, which will reduce the stress in your life.

Plan a vacation

You can limit it to a staycation weekend, or a hunting trip, the point is that it doesn't have to be an expensive week in the tropics with a ton of friends or family. Just the process of planning a vacation and having something to look forward to can improve your mood for as much as eight weeks, according to mental health experts.

Concentrate on your strengths

To curtail stress, it is best to start your day with things you are good at, because that will build your confidence. Tackle tougher tasks later in the day.

Try new things

Writing poems, painting, or trying hiking—engaging in new activities will make it easier to overcome stress and anxiety because they will lift your mood. Also, creative expression and overall health are linked.

How Does Self-help Affect Mental Health?

The term "self-care" has become more popular recently. There are many products, services, and health professionals that promote the practice of self-care. However, many people don't actually know how to describe self-care, and how it affects our mental health.

In this section, we shall look at the role self-care plays in our mental health, and how you can use it to take care of yourself—both mentally and physically.

Self-care is not a new idea, and it is not complex or exclusive. Self-care is simply described as taking care of yourself. At its core, it comprises conscious steps that preserve or improve our mental or physical well-being. It is all about taking deliberate steps to engage in activities that look after you and your health.

What do studies reveal about self-care and mental health? Since self-care is the practice of caring for the physical, emotional, and psychological well-being of a person, it shouldn't be a surprise that it affects your mental health. Self-care depends on increased self-awareness, which is beneficial to those suffering from mental illness. The practice of cultivating self-awareness can help you identify patterns in your feelings and cope with events or situations that can lead to worsened symptoms. Self-awareness can also help you recognize the activities necessary for your well-being, soothe negative symptoms of mental illness, and leave you feeling more pleased with yourself.

Listing examples of self-care strategies is not an easy thing to do. The truth is, self–care is not the same for any two people you meet! For example, extroverted people see being around others in a social gathering to satisfy their emotional needs, but introverts prefer a quiet evening spent watching a movie with a close friend or a spouse to meet their social needs. Then there are some who enjoy warm bubble baths, facial masks, and slow music.

Consequently, others see engaging in strenuous activities, such as exercise, as a coping mechanism. Drinking coffee with a friend, taking a vacation, fishing, and hunting are also examples of self-care for many people.

There is no limit to the way you can practice self-care, and in the end, all that matters is that you do what you enjoy most. Although some people think that pampering themselves or participating in guilty pleasures is the best way to enjoy self-care, it goes beyond that. Self-care comprises all the things necessary to remain healthy, curtail stress, and feel as mentally balanced as possible. Therefore, getting a massage and cleaning your home to lessen stress can all be a part of your self-care. Enjoying an ice cream on a hot day qualifies as self-care, as does attending a therapy session to discuss your emotional needs, trauma, or mental illness.

You may already be doing something to manage your symptoms. If you want to do more, then keep in mind that self-care doesn't need to be elaborate, costly, or labor-intensive to be effective. Creating a list of your favorite self-care strategies can help you recognize what activities suit you best, improve your mood, or help you reduce stress. A written list can benefit you by helping you promptly decide what to do when you feel overwhelmed. The style of self-care you practice will depend on what you really need, enjoy, and your energy levels. In addition, personality and other related factors play a vital role in choosing self-care methods. Here are some common self-care ideas that will get you started:

Carry out a rapid mental survey of your body

It is best to do this when breathing deeply. Scan your entire body, and release tension as you find it. Assess your posture and change it if necessary. You only need a few seconds to complete this mental survey, but the processes can yield instant results.

Maintain healthy sleep habits and listen to your body

Going to bed early, making your bedroom as comfortable and quiet as possible, and practicing good screen-time habits before bed will all enable you to enjoy a more peaceful sleep.

Pay attention to your health needs, and take care of them

A perfect example of how to take care of your health is attending regularly scheduled appointments with your doctor. Along with those checkups, follow a strict regimen of prescribed medication, go for therapy appointments, chiropractic adjustments, or any other care necessary for your overall health.

Listen to your favorite music or watch a movie

Music is therapeutic! Listening to music, or watching a movie are great examples of self-care. For introverted people, sitting at home in the evening and watching a movie is an excellent way to improve their mood.

Create a list of five or more things you like about your-self

Many people have a low opinion of themselves. Low self-esteem is a major trigger for stress and anxiety. To improve your self-esteem, create a list of at least five things you like about yourself. This list will help you feel good about yourself. Although it may feel like a small gesture, it can do wonders for your self-confidence.

Make time for a skincare routine, if it helps

Having a beauty or skincare routine can improve many people's moods, especially women. If you are one of these people, set aside time to pamper yourself often! The difference this will make in your overall mental health may surprise you!

Allocate time to talk to a friend or a therapist

Many people find it beneficial to talk to someone about their feelings. You can speak to a close friend, family member, or a therapist. Alternatively, you can journal, read self-help books, or quietly reflect on your day.

If there's no one around you can speak to, there is always yourself! Many people say they feel better after having a conversation within themselves. It will also increase self-awareness, which is an essential part of self-care, but many people ignore it.

Don't agree to something you don't want to do

Learn to say "no" to something you don't like or want to do. Agreeing to take on too many tasks, or being responsible for too many things at once, can cause you extreme stress and anxiety, because you cannot give your all to everything at once! If you take on too many tasks at the same time, then you won't succeed in all of them, and this will dampen your confidence.

Why is Self-care Important?

I know I might be repeating myself, but this is one of the things that got me through my grief. Self-care is an essential part of living a healthy and happy life. Paying attention to yourself, both mentally and physically, is vital to taking control of your overall health. Most of us live extremely busy lives. This is why we tend to forget about ourselves, especially those of us with multiple responsibilities and other people we cater to in our lives. If this describes you, then keep in mind that looking after yourself will improve your wellbeing, and the better you feel, the better you will be at taking care of others. Self-care is about committing to putting yourself first, even if it is for a short time.

All of this doesn't mean that self-care is the cure for mental or physical illnesses, although self-care can undeniably help people with mental or physical illnesses. Research has also revealed that many people fail to offer themselves sufficient self-care amidst the stress of dealing with their symptoms. Most people find it hard to practice self-care when it is most necessary, like in times of fatigue, or when feeling despair. Some will also feel a sense of guilt for participating in something pleasurable, or feel unable to due to pain, immobility, or other reasons. Many well-meaning people speak about the benefits of self-care to those suffering from depression, anxiety, stress, and other mental or physical illnesses, but these people rarely recognize the amount of effort needed for self-care, or the struggles of people who are trying to care for themselves while suffering from symptoms of mental illness.

Benefits of Self-Care

There are lots of benefits associated with self-care—most of which are interlinked—and they combine and compound to enhance your overall well-being.

Self-care boosts physical health

A significant part of self-care is committing to looking after your body and becoming more attuned to your physical needs. For example, brushing your teeth regularly, exercising more, or spending time with your loved ones. Whatever it looks like for you, a part of your self-care strategy should focus on looking after your physical health needs.

Self-care improves self-esteem

Practicing self-care involves treating yourself with kindness, and this will make you love and respect yourself more. It will also help you calm your nerves and provide more time to look after yourself. This will all boost your self-esteem. Surveys by mental health experts reveal that people with good self-esteem find it easier to overcome setbacks and have better chances of meeting their goals.

Self-care reduces stress and anxiety

Set aside time for relaxing activities, such as meditation. Watching your favorite movie is a great example of this! These activities are known to reduce symptoms of stress and anxiety.

Self-care can help build better relationships

If you think about it, you won't be surprised—the happier and healthier a person is, the more they can commit to a relationship. For this reason, it is even more crucial that parents or guardians rigorously practice self-care.

Section Five:

LEAP OF FAITH

Life is about taking important steps in pursuit of your aims. The most difficult decision to make is actually deciding on what to do next and then doing it! Even though you may have identified the root cause of your problems, understood it, and realized that support/help is crucial, you still have to take a leap of faith. As discussed in the previous chapter, therapy can help. Share what you feel with your health professionals, because the fact is, they are in the best position to help you overcome your mental health issues. Don't settle for a mental health professional that is not the best fit for you. Keep looking until you find one that works for you.

I've always imagined myself to be the Superman that can take on anything. Because Superman is one of the strongest superheroes—not just in DC, but in all comics. I have always likened myself to him. Why? Because I am the one who helps people and has lived through and seen a lot of traumas. I thought I didn't have a limit, and that I wouldn't be affected by these things. But the thing about Superman is that he is alone and has no one to go to with his problems. He doesn't have anyone who can relate to him. Would he ask the lady he just saved how to deal with the weight of the world on his shoulders? Nope. So, sometimes Superman gets tired, burnt out, and feels like giving up.

I didn't realize I was in that place until I fell back into my PTSD when my son passed away in 2016. Then came the death of my father in 2018. I didn't develop PTSD just because of those things, but the memory of the loss of my child contributed to not being able to hold things together anymore. There came a point when I couldn't hold it all in anymore.

However, I didn't give up. I took a leap of faith and sought help from support groups, counseling, and the Wounded Warrior Project. I was finally able to overcome my PTSD again, with the help of all those things that combined to form my very own Justice League. Superman has the Justice League to talk to, and you have us.

We may not suffer the way he does, but we all have our own pain to deal with, and that pain can be overwhelming at times. We tend to find ourselves avoiding things we think will cause us harm or make us uncomfortable. This can look like avoiding new job opportunities, career advancements, relationships, social situations, recreational activities, and family get-togethers. Someone once told me that at least they know and understand the pain they are feeling now, so they didn't want to take a chance and step into something they aren't familiar with. People use avoidance as a natural coping mechanism for pain, trauma, and other mental health issues.

It is wise to avoid dangerous situations or peer pressure, but avoidance is more than just not wanting to feel uncomfortable. Avoiding something can make you feel in control. However, depending on what you are avoiding, it doesn't always signify true control. Long-term, these behaviors can exacerbate other issues going on in your life. Most feel shame in doing this and call it procrastination. Procrastination is defined as to put something off intentionally and habitually. The word "procrastinate" originates from the Latin prefix pro-, meaning "forward," and *crastinus*, "of tomorrow." The word means moving or acting slowly, to fall behind, and it implies blameworthy delay, especially through laziness or apathy. It's the self-blaming that gets us in trouble.

Procrastination is one of the most common ways people avoid their problems. But what if there was a way to get through it?

Here are five steps to help you overcome procrastination:

1. Make a list of your favorite avoidance behaviors (computer games, cookies, TV, shopping, addictions, etc.).

2. Whenever you think of doing the behavior, or find yourself doing it, ask yourself: "What am I avoiding?"

3. Think about the thing you're avoiding and notice what you're feeling (anxiety, frustration, daunted). Stay with that feeling.

4. Then, just do the thing! If you can do it right away, great! If not, make a definite plan for a set time and feel those feelings while also doing what needs to be done.

5. Reward yourself when it's done! You can use harmless things on your avoidance list as reinforcers once the task is complete.

Make that decision and don't procrastinate. Like the old adage says, procrastination is dangerous, so don't suffer alone. Share your pains with a medical doctor, with a family member, a friend, or a therapist. Let everyone know what you are feeling deep inside. That important step might just save you from a total collapse. So, make that decision and never give up. The sun will always shine again, and the grass will turn green.

Conclusion

If you're suffering from a mental disorder, you're not alone.

You're not alone in your suffering, and you're not alone in your hope for recovery. There are millions of us around the globe who have struggled or who are struggling with mental illness. And there are millions more who know someone who is or has.

This book is for those who suffer from a mental health disorder and their loved ones. It's important for family and friends to understand that treating a mental disorder is more than just going to see the doctor for sessions. Support from family and friends is essential to recovery. I hope this book teaches you that.

Mental health issues are common, but solutions are available. You can get better during treatment and recover entirely. First, you must comprehend the five elements to your path of recovery—awareness, understanding your problem, perception, support, and taking a leap of faith.

Having a mental disorder isn't the end of the world. Help is out there and is more abundant now with all the awareness programs and empowerment organizations across the world. Hopefully, this book has helped you to identify some of the best ways you can cope with your mental illness. You, too, can become a better person and live the wonderful life that was destined for you!